Multi-Perspective Management of Sleep Disorders

Editors

AMANDA J. PIPER
STEPHEN MCNAMARA
BRENDON J. YEE

SLEEP MEDICINE CLINICS

www.sleep.theclinics.com

September 2024 • Volume 19 • Number 3

ELSEVIER

1600 John F. Kennedy Boulevard • Suite 1800 • Philadelphia, Pennsylvania, 19103-2899

http://www.theclinics.com

SLEEP MEDICINE CLINICS Volume 19, Number 3
September 2024, ISSN 1556-407X, ISBN-13: 978-0-443-29374-0

Editor: Joanna Gascoine
Developmental Editor: Akshay Samson

Sleep Medicine Clinics (ISSN 1556-407X) is published quarterly by Elsevier Inc., 360 Park Avenue South, New York, NY 10010-1710. Months of issue are March, June, September and December. Business and Editorial Offices: 1600 John F. Kennedy Blvd., Ste. 1800, Philadelphia, PA 19103-2899. Customer Service Office: 3251 Riverport Lane, Maryland Heights, MO 63043. Periodicals postage paid at New York, NY and additional mailing offices. Subscription prices are $246.00 per year (US individuals), $100.00 (US and Canadian students), $283.00 (Canadian individuals), $292.00 (international individuals) $135.00 (International students). For institutional access pricing please contact Customer Service via the contact information below. Foreign air speed delivery is included in all *Clinics* subscription prices. All prices are subject to change without notice. Orders, claims, and journal inquiries: Please visit our Support Hub page https://service.elsevier.com for assistance.

Reprints. For copies of 100 or more of articles in this publication, please contact the Commercial Reprints Department, Elsevier Inc., 360 Park Avenue South, New York, NY 10010-1710. Tel.: 212-633-3874; Fax: 212-633-3820; E-mail: reprints@elsevier.com.

Sleep Medicine Clinics is covered in *MEDLINE/PubMed (Index Medicus)*.

SLEEP MEDICINE CLINICS

ISSUES OF RELATED INTEREST

Neurologic Clinics
https://www.neurologic.theclinics.com/

THE CLINICS ARE AVAILABLE ONLINE!
Access your subscription at:
www.theclinics.com

Contributors

CONSULTING EDITORS

TEOFILO LEE-CHIONG Jr, MD
Professor of Medicine, National Jewish Health, Professor of Medicine, University of Colorado, Denver, Colorado, USA; Chief Medical Liaison, Philips Respironics, Murrysville, Pennsylvania, USA

DIEGO GARCIA-BORREGUERO, MD, PhD
International Medical Director Instituto del Sueño, Calle Padre Damián, Madrid, Spain

ANA C. KRIEGER, MD, MPH, FCCP, FAASM
Chief, Division of Sleep Neurology, Medical Director, Weill Cornell Center for Sleep Medicine, Professor of Clinical Medicine, Professor of Medicine in Neurology and Genetic Medicine, Weill Cornell Medical College, Cornell University, New York, New York, USA

EDITORS

AMANDA J. PIPER, BAppSc (Phty), MEd, PhD
Clinical Lead, Department of Respiratory and Sleep Medicine, Respiratory Support Service, Royal Prince Alfred Hospital, Faculty of Medicine and Health, University of Sydney, Camperdown, New South Wales, Australia

STEPHEN McNAMARA, BSc (Med), MBBS, PhD
Senior Staff Specialist, Department of Respiratory and Sleep Medicine, Royal Prince Alfred Hospital, Faculty of Medicine and Health, University of Sydney, Camperdown, New South Wales, Australia

BRENDON J. YEE, MBChB, FRACP, PhD
Clinical Professor, Department of Respiratory and Sleep Medicine, Royal Prince Alfred Hospital, Head, Discipline of Sleep Medicine, Sydney Medical School, University of Sydney, Camperdown, New South Wales, Australia; Honarary Professor, Woolcock Institute of Medical Research, Sleep and Circadian Research Group, Macquarie University, Sydney, New South Wales, Australia

AUTHORS

RESHMA AMIN, MD, MSc
Pediatric Respirologist, Division of Respiratory Medicine, The Hospital for Sick Children, University of Toronto, Toronto, Ontario, Canada

TIINA ANDERSEN, BSc(Hons), MSc, PhD
Associate Professor, The Department of Health and Functioning, Western Norway University of Applied Science, Postdoctoral Research Fellow, Thoracic Department, Haukeland University Hospital, Bergen, Norway

JEAN-MICHEL ARNAL, MD
Senior Intensivist, Service de Réanimation Polyvalente et Unité de Ventilation à Domicile, Hôpital Sainte Musse, Toulon, France

GERRIE BLADDER, RN
Specialised Respiratory Nurse, Department of Pulmonary Diseases, Home Mechanical Ventilation, University of Groningen, University Medical Center Groningen, Groningen, the Netherlands

MICHELLE CHATWIN, BSc(Hons), PhD
Consultant Physiotherapist, NMCC, The National Hospital for Neurology and Neurosurgery, University College London Hospitals Foundation Trust, Clinical and Academic Department of Sleep and Breathing, Royal Brompton Hospital, Part of Guys and St Thomas' NHS Foundation Trust, London, United Kingdom

MARIEKE L. DUIVERMAN, MD, PhD
Assistant Professor, Department of Pulmonary Diseases, Home Mechanical Ventilation, University of Groningen, University Medical Center Groningen, Groningen, the Netherlands

Dr EMMA GRAY, MBBS (Hons), FRACP, MPH
Respiratory and Sleep Physician, Department of Respiratory and Sleep Medicine, Royal Prince Alfred Hospital, Central Clinical Medical School, The University of Sydney, Camperdown, New South Wales, Australia

LESLEY HOWARD, BAppSc (Physiotherapy), MHlthSc (Cardiopulmonary Physiotherapy)
Senior Physiotherapist, Department of Respiratory and Sleep Medicine, Westmead Hospital, Western Sydney Local Health District, Westmead, New South Wales, Australia

FILIPA JESUS, MD
Resident, Pulmonology Department, Unidade Local de Saúde da Guarda EPE, Guarda, Portugal; Department of Pulmonary Diseases, Home Mechanical Ventilation, University of Groningen, University Medical Center Groningen, Groningen, the Netherlands

SONIA KHIRANI, PhD
Researcher, ASV Santé, Gennevilliers, France; AP-HP Hôpital Necker-Enfants maladies, Unité de ventilation non-invasive et sommeil, Paris, France

STEPHEN McNAMARA, BSc (Med), MBBS, PhD
Senior Staff Specialist, Department of Respiratory and Sleep Medicine, Royal Prince Alfred Hospital, Camperdown, New South Wales, Australia

COLLETTE MENADUE, BAppSc(Phty), PhD
Senior Physiotherapist, Department of Respiratory and Sleep Medicine, Royal Prince Alfred Hospital, Camperdown, New South Wales, Australia

PATRICK B. MURPHY, MBBS, PhD, MRCP
Consultant, Lane Fox Respiratory Service, Division of Heart, Lung and Critical Care, Guy's and St Thomas NHS Foundation Trust, St Thomas' Hospital, Reader in Respiratory Medicine, King's College London, Strand, London, United Kingdom

BUDHIMA NANAYAKKARA, MBBS, PhB
Associate Professor of Medicine, Charles Sturt University, Staff Specialist in Respiratory, Sleep and General Medicine, Orange Health Service, Orange, New South Wales, Australia

BENJAMIN H.M. NGUYEN, BSc (Hons), MBBS, FRACP
Director of Respiratory Failure Service, Department of Thoracic Medicine, St Vincent's Hospital, Sydney, New South Wales, Australia; Visiting Medical Officer, Department of Respiratory and Sleep Medicine, Royal Prince Alfred Hospital, Clinical Lecturer, Sydney Medical School, Sydney University, Camperdown, New South Wales, Australia; Woolcock Institute of Medical Research, Macquarie University, Macquarie Park, New South Wales, Australia

MAXIME PATOUT, MD
Clinical Expert, AP-HP, Groupe Hospitalier Universitaire AP-HP-Sorbonne Université, site Pitié-Salpêtrière, Service des Pathologies du Sommeil (Département R3S), Sorbonne Université, INSERM, UMRS1158 Neurophysiologie Respiratoire Expérimentale et Clinique, Paris, France

AMANDA J. PIPER, BAppSc (Phty), MEd, PhD
Clinical Lead, Department of Respiratory and Sleep Medicine, Respiratory Support Service, Royal Prince Alfred Hospital, Faculty of Medicine and Health, University of Sydney, Camperdown, New South Wales, Australia

MARY M. ROBERTS, MSN, BHS, MSPC, DipAppSc(Nursing)
Clinical Nurse Consultant, Department of Respiratory and Sleep Medicine, Westmead Hospital, Western Sydney Local Health District, Faculty of Medicine and Health, The University of Sydney, Faculty of Medicine and Health, Westmead Clinical School, Ludwig Engel Centre for Respiratory Research, Westmead Institute for Medical Research, Westmead, New South Wales, Australia; Faculty of Health, Improving Palliative Care, Aged and Chronic Care through Clinical Research and Translation (IMPACCT), University of Technology, Ultimo, New South Wales, Australia

ALFREDO SELIM, MD, MPH
Assistant Professor of Medicine, Department of Emergency Medicine, Boston University School of Medicine, Veterans Affairs Medical Center, West Roxbury, Massachusetts, USA

BERNARDO SELIM, MD
Associate Professor of Medicine, Division of Pulmonary and Critical Care Medicine, Mayo Clinic Alix School of Medicine, Director of the Respiratory Care Unit, Mayo Clinic Center for Sleep Medicine, Mayo Clinic, Rochester, Minnesota, USA

NICOLE L. SHEERS, BPhysio(Hons), MPhysio, PhD
Postdoctoral Research Fellow, Department of Physiotherapy, Melbourne School of Health Sciences, The University of Melbourne, Parkville, Victoria, Australia; The Institute for Breathing and Sleep, Austin Health, Heidelberg, Victoria, Australia

TRACY A. SMITH, BSc, MBBS, PhD
Staff Specialist, Department of Respiratory and Sleep Medicine, Westmead Hospital, Western Sydney Local Health District, The University of Sydney, Faculty of Medicine and Health, Westmead Clinical School, Westmead, New South Wales, Australia

XINHANG TU, MB
Fellow Physician, Division of Pulmonary and Critical Care Medicine, Mayo Clinic Center for Sleep Medicine, Mayo Clinic, Rochester, Minnesota, USA

PETER J. WIJKSTRA, MD, PhD
Professor, Department of Pulmonary Diseases, Home Mechanical Ventilation, University of Groningen, University Medical Center Groningen, Groningen, the Netherlands

LENA XIAO, MD, MSc
Pediatric Respirologist, Division of Respiratory Medicine, British Columbia Children's Hospital, University of British Columbia, Vancouver, British Columbia, Canada

BRENDON J. YEE, MBChB, FRACP, PhD
Clinical Professor, Department of Respiratory and Sleep Medicine, Royal Prince Alfred Hospital, Camperdown, New South Wales, Australia; Head, Discipline of Sleep Medicine, Sydney Medical School, University of Sydney, Camperdown, New South Wales, Australia; Honarary Professor, Woolcock Institute of Medical Research, Sleep and Circadian Research Group, Macquarie University, Sydney, New South Wales, Australia

Contents

issue, provided that it is a comfortable, safe environment in which adequate monitoring can be assured. The majority of patients prefer their own home for treatment initiation.

Interfaces for Home Noninvasive Ventilation

Amanda J. Piper

The choice of interface used to deliver noninvasive ventilation (NIV) is a critical element in successfully and safely establishing home NIV in people with sleep hypoventilation syndromes. Both patient-related and equipment-related factors need to be considered when selecting an interface. Recognizing specific issues that can occur with a particular style of mask is important when troubleshooting NIV problems and attempting to minimize side effects. Access to a range of mask styles and designs to use on a rotational basis is especially important for patients using NIV on a more continuous basis, those at risk of developing pressure areas, and children.

Telemonitoring in Non-invasive Ventilation

Sonia Khirani, Maxime Patout, and Jean-Michel Arnal

Telemonitoring in non-invasive ventilation is constantly evolving to enable follow-up of adults and children. Depending on the device and manufacturer, different ventilator variables are displayed on web-based platforms. However, high-granularity measurement is not always available remotely, which precludes breath-by-breath waveforms and precise monitoring of nocturnal gas exchange. Therefore, telemonitoring is mainly useful for monitoring utilization of the device, leaks, and respiratory events. Coordinated relationships between patients, homecare providers, and hospital teams are necessary to transform available data into diagnosis and actions. Telemonitoring is time and cost-consuming. The balance between cost, workload, and clinical benefit should be further evaluated.

The Role of High Flow Nasal Therapy in Chronic Respiratory Failure

Emma Gray and Collette Menadue

High-flow nasal therapy (HFNT) has an increasing role in the management of acute hypoxic respiratory failure. Due to its tolerable interface and ease of use, its role in chronic hypercapnic respiratory failure (CHRF) is emerging. This article examines the literature to date surrounding the short and long-term mechanisms of HFNT in sleep and wakefulness of CHRF patients. It is likely HFNT will have an increasing role in those patients intolerant of non-invasive ventilation.

Impact of Disease-modifying Therapies on Respiratory Function in People with Neuromuscular Disorders

Lena Xiao and Reshma Amin

Spinal muscular atrophy (SMA) and Duchenne muscular dystrophy (DMD) are neuromuscular disorders that affect muscular function. The most common causes of morbidity and mortality are respiratory complications, including restrictive lung disease, ineffective cough, and sleep-disordered breathing. The paradigm of care is changing as new disease-modifying therapies are altering disease trajectory, outcomes, expectations, as well as patient and caregiver experiences. This article provides an overview on therapeutic advances for SMA and DMD in the last 10 years, with a focus on the effects of disease-modifying therapies on respiratory function.

High-quality respiratory care and airway clearance is essential for people with neuro-muscular disease (pwNMD) as respiratory tract infections are a major cause of morbidity and mortality. This review expands on published guidelines by highlighting the role of cough peak flow along with other options for cough evaluation, and discusses recent key research findings which have influenced the practice of respiratory therapy for pwNMD.

Palliative care is important for many patients who require noninvasive ventilation. The particular needs of patients with neuromuscular disease and chronic obstructive pulmonary disease are explored. Advance care planning is explored with tips for undertaking this important communication task. Brief comments regarding symptom burden, weaning, voluntary assisted dying, and self-care are included.

Preface

Updates on Chronic Respiratory Failure and Noninvasive Respiratory Support: Innovations and Insights

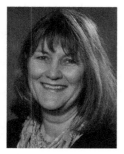

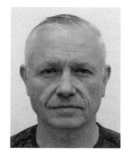

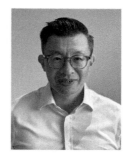

Amanda J. Piper, BAppSc (Phty), MEd, PhD

Stephen McNamara, BSc (Med), MBBS, PhD

Brendon J. Yee, MBChB, PhD

Editors

It has been almost 40 years since the use of nocturnal nasal noninvasive ventilation (NIV) was first described by Ellis, Sullivan and colleagues,[1–3] who demonstrated the feasibility and effectiveness of the technique in normalizing nocturnal breathing in patients with neuromuscular and chest wall disorders. Other forms of nocturnal ventilatory support had been used prior to this to manage chronic hypercapnic respiratory failure, including cuirass ventilators, mouthpiece ventilation, and tracheostomy.[4,5] However, the number of individuals managed using these earlier techniques remained low, and only a small number of specialized centers offered these therapies. The ease with which NIV could be applied, the high rate of treatment acceptance, and its obvious clinical and subjective benefits encouraged the widespread use of nocturnal NIV, and within a few years, a broader range of disorders was shown to respond favorably to therapy.[6–8]

In this collection of articles, the mechanisms by which events during sleep can result in the development of awake respiratory failure (article in this issue, "Pathophysiology of Chronic Hypercapnic Respiratory Failure," by Nanayakka and McNamara), and

the types of clinical assessment clinicians should employ to identify individuals at risk of sleep hypoventilation (article in this issue, "Assessment of Chronic Hypercapnic Respiratory Failure," by Tu and colleagues) are reviewed. An under-appreciated condition commonly associated with chronic respiratory failure, the Overlap Syndrome (article in this issue, "Chronic Obstructive Pulmonary Disease and Obstructive Sleep Apnea Overlap Syndrome: An Update on the Epidemiology, Pathophysiology, and Management" by Nguyen and colleagues) is featured in this issue. An earlier issue of *Sleep Medicine Clinics* comprehensively covered other conditions amenable to home NIV, and the reader is encouraged to review this work.[9] Despite improvements in mask and device technology, management of chronic respiratory failure with NIV can be challenging at times. The interface used to link the patient to the ventilator is a key element in achieving positive outcomes with NIV (article in this issue, "Interfaces for Home Noninvasive Ventilation," by Piper) and is a major consideration in initiating NIV (article in this issue, "Initiation of Chronic Noninvasive Ventilation," by Duiverman and colleagues). Improvements in ventilator technology are providing

Sleep Med Clin 19 (2024) xiii–xv
https://doi.org/10.1016/j.jsmc.2024.06.001
1556-407X/24/© 2024 Published by Elsevier Inc.

the opportunity to offer more effective therapy, and importantly, monitor this therapy remotely with the goal of optimizing ventilation. However, much more work is needed to better understand how to translate these data into improved work processes and clinical outcomes (article in this issue, "Telemonitoring in Noninvasive Ventilation," by Khirani and colleagues).

Managing chronic respiratory failure in the home does not end with NIV. Other articles in this series explore potential therapy options beyond or in addition to NIV. There is increasing interest and research into medications able to influence the natural history of neuromuscular disorders (article in this issue, "Impact of Disease-modifying Therapies on Respiratory Function in People with Neuromuscular Disorders," by Xiao and Amin), with the aim of delaying or preventing the development of disability, including respiratory failure. Despite our best efforts, not all individuals will accept and tolerate NIV. High-flow nasal therapy is emerging as a potential adjunct or alternative to NIV in selected patients with respiratory failure requiring home therapy (article in this issue, "The Role of HighFlow Nasal Therapy in Chronic Respiratory Failure," by Gray and Menadue). While NIV can effectively reverse respiratory failure in those with respiratory muscle weakness, poor cough effectiveness with retention of secretions is a major source of morbidity and mortality. Although the evidence base for airway clearance techniques in people with respiratory muscle weakness is still evolving, understanding the principles of producing an effective cough and clearance of retained secretions is fundamental in identifying what techniques to use in different circumstances (article in this issue, "Airway Clearance in Neuromuscular Disease," by Sheers and colleagues). The importance of viewing palliative care as part of the comprehensive management of chronic respiratory failure, rather than a process simply addressing end of life care, is also highlighted (article in this issue, "Palliative Care and Noninvasive Ventilation," by Smith and colleagues).

We are now standing on the cusp of an exciting future in home ventilation. As in other areas of medicine, artificial intelligence systems along with large data networks have the potential to transform the home ventilation landscape over the next few decades. No matter what changes are in store, we must always place the patient and their needs at the center of our care processes.

We are truly grateful to each of the contributors for their time and insights into these pertinent topics. We also thank *Sleep Medicine Clinics* for giving us the opportunity to be part of this issue.

DISCLOSURES

AP has received honoraria for educational activities presented on behalf of ResMed Asia-Pacific and Philips, manufacturers of consumables and positive pressure devices designed for sleep disordered breathing.

Amanda J. Piper, BAppSc (Phty), MEd, PhD
Department of Respiratory and
Sleep Medicine
Royal Prince Alfred Hospital
Camperdown, New South Wales 2050, Australia

Faculty of Medicine and Health
University of Sydney
Sydney, New South Wales, Australia

Stephen McNamara, BSc (Med), MBBS, PhD
Department of Respiratory and
Sleep Medicine
Royal Prince Alfred Hospital
Camperdown, New South Wales 2050, Australia

Faculty of Medicine and Health
University of Sydney
Sydney, New South Wales, Australia

Brendon J. Yee, MBChB, PhD
Department of Respiratory and
Sleep Medicine
Royal Prince Alfred Hospital
Camperdown, New South Wales 2050, Australia

Discipline of Sleep Medicine
Sydney Medical School
University of Sydney
New South Wales, Australia

Woolcock Institute of Medical Research
Sleep and Circadian Research Group
Macquarie University
Sydney, New South Wales 2109, Australia

E-mail addresses:
Amanda.Piper@health.nsw.gov.au (A.J. Piper)
Stephen.McNamara1@health.nsw.gov.au
(S. McNamara)
Brendon.Yee@health.nsw.gov.au (B.J. Yee)

REFERENCES

1. Ellis ER, Bye PT, Bruderer JW, et al. Treatment of respiratory failure during sleep in patients with neuromuscular disease. Positive-pressure ventilation through a nose mask. Am Rev Respir Dis 1987;135(1):148–52.

2. Sullivan CE, Ellis ER. Nocturnal positive pressure ventilation via a nasal mask. Am Rev Respir Dis 1987;136(3):791–2.

3. Ellis ER, Grunstein RR, Chan S, et al. Noninvasive ventilatory support during sleep improves respiratory failure in kyphoscoliosis. Chest 1988;94(4): 811–5.

4. Collier CR, Affeldt JE. Ventilatory efficiency of the cuirass respirator in totally paralyzed chronic poliomyelitis patients. J Appl Physiol 1954;6(9): 531–8.

5. Bach JR, Alba AS, Saporito LR. Intermittent positive pressure ventilation via the mouth as an alternative to tracheostomy for 257 ventilator users. Chest 1993;103:174–82.

6. Hodson ME, Madden BP, Steven MH, et al. Non-invasive mechanical ventilation for cystic fibrosis patients—a potential bridge to transplantation. Eur Respir J 1991;4(5):524–7.

7. Piper AJ, Sullivan CE. Effects of short-term NIPPV in the treatment of patients with severe obstructive sleep apnea and hypercapnia. Chest 1994;105(2): 434–40.

8. Windisch W, Vogel M, Sorichter S, et al. Normocapnia during nIPPV in chronic hypercapnic COPD reduces subsequent spontaneous PaCO2. Respir Med 2002; 96(8):572–9.

9. Wolfe LF, Sergew A. Non-invasive ventilation. Sleep Med Clin 2020;15(4):i–598.

Pathophysiology of Chronic Hypercapnic Respiratory Failure

Budhima Nanayakkara, MBBS, PhB[a,b,c,]*,
Stephen McNamara, BSc(Med), MBBS, PhD[d,1]

KEYWORDS

- Chronic hypercapnic respiratory failure • Hypoventilation syndromes • Control of breathing
- Respiratory physiology • Oxygen-induced hypercapnia • Load-capacity balance
- Nocturnal hypoventilation

KEY POINTS

- Chronic hypercapnic respiratory failure (CHRF) occurs due to chronic alveolar hypoventilation with respect to metabolic carbon dioxide (CO_2) production.
- Multiple mechanisms contribute to the development of CHRF, including the interplay of any derangements that abnormally increase metabolic CO_2 production, reduce minute ventilation ($V'e$), or increase dead space fraction (Vd/VT).
- Sleep-related hypoventilation is very common and contributes to the development of diurnal hypercapnia through bicarbonate retention and cerebrospinal fluid alkalosis.
- Patients with CHRF are sensitive to hyperoxia, mostly from a combination of worsening ventilation/ perfusion mismatch and increased Vd/Vt.

INTRODUCTION

The major task of the respiratory system is to maintain adequate gas exchange, ensuring sufficient oxygenation to fuel aerobic respiration while simultaneously maintaining a steady state blood carbon dioxide (CO_2) tension.[1] Failure to accomplish this leads to respiratory failure.

Respiratory failure is broadly categorized into 2 types. Type 1 (or hypoxemic) respiratory failure is defined when arterial oxygen (O_2) tensions are abnormally low, by convention less than 60 mm Hg, accompanied by a normal range or low arterial CO_2 tension (<45 mm Hg). Type 2 (or hypercapnic) respiratory failure occurs when arterial CO_2 tensions are abnormally elevated (>45 mm Hg). Hypercapnic respiratory failure is further classified by chronicity as

being acute, chronic, or acute-on-chronic. Chronic hypercapnic respiratory failure (CHRF) is almost always secondary to alveolar hypoventilation, and unless the patient is on supplemental oxygen, is frequently accompanied by arterial hypoxemia.

This review will focus on the pathogenesis of CHRF, with a particular emphasis on the role sleep plays in contributing to the vulnerability of respiration in these conditions.

THE PHYSIOLOGIC DETERMINANTS OF ARTERIAL CARBON DIOXIDE

Metabolic production of CO_2 ($V'CO_2$) occurs predominantly through substrate flux via the Krebs cycle,[2] while the elimination of CO_2 occurs via ventilation (**Fig. 1**).

[a] Charles Sturt University, 346 Leeds Parade, Orange, NSW 2800, Australia; [b] Department of Medicine, Orange Health Service, Orange, NSW 2800, Australia; [c] University of Sydney, Camperdown, NSW 2006, Australia; [d] Department of Respiratory & Sleep Medicine, Royal Prince Alfred Hospital, Camperdown, NSW 2050, Australia
[1] Present address: Department of Respiratory & Sleep Medicine, Royal Prince Alfred Hospital, Camperdown, NSW 2050, Australia.
* Corresponding author. Charles Sturt University, 346 Leeds Parade, Orange, NSW 2800, Australia
E-mail addresses: Budhima.nanayakkar@health.nsw.gov.au; Budhima.nanayakkara@gmail.com

Sleep Med Clin 19 (2024) 379–389
https://doi.org/10.1016/j.jsmc.2024.04.001

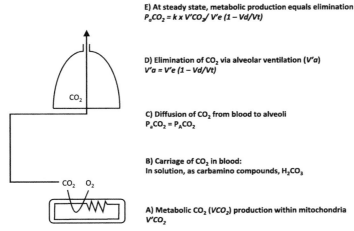

E) At steady state, metabolic production equals elimination
$P_aCO_2 = k \times V'CO_2 / V'e\ (1 - Vd/Vt)$

D) Elimination of CO_2 via alveolar ventilation ($V'a$)
$V'a = V'e\ (1 - Vd/Vt)$

C) Diffusion of CO_2 from blood to alveoli
$P_aCO_2 = P_ACO_2$

B) Carriage of CO_2 in blood:
In solution, as carbamino compounds, H_2CO_3

A) Metabolic CO_2 (VCO_2) production within mitochondria
$V'CO_2$

Fig. 1. CO_2 production occurs in the mitochondria, through the Krebs cycle. CO_2 diffuses into the systemic capillaries and is carried by blood in solution as carbamino compounds and as carbonic acid (H_2CO_3). At the level of the pulmonary capillaries, CO_2 diffuses into the alveoli passively, governed by Fick's law of diffusion. There is usually complete equilibration between pulmonary capillary (arterial) CO_2 ($Paco_2$) and alveolar CO_2 (P_ACO_2). While elimination of CO_2 occurs via alveolar ventilation ($V'a$), only perfused alveoli participate in CO_2 clearance. In steady state, elimination of CO_2 via alveolar ventilation equals $V'CO_2$, whereby $Paco_2 = k \times V'CO_2/V'e\ (1 - Vd/Vt)$, where $V'e$ is the total ventilation, Vd is the dead space volume, and Vt is the tidal volume.

Total ventilation ($V'e$) is the product of respiratory rate (f) and tidal volume (Vt), with the Vt consisting of alveolar volume (Va) plus the volume of gas that does not participate in gas exchange (dead space volume: Vd). It follows that CHRF may thus result from either one of or, more commonly, a combination of factors that result in an elevated arterial CO_2 (P_aco_2) including conditions that (1) increase metabolic production of CO_2; (2) decrease $V'e$; and/or (3) increase the Vd (expressed physiologically as an increased dead space fraction: Vd/Vt).[3]

Ventilation/perfusion (V/Q) mismatch is by far the commonest mechanism of hypoxemic respiratory failure. However, despite low V/Q regions contributing to increases in end capillary CO_2, the net effect of increased P_aco_2 is to signal an increase in $V'e$ via chemoreception. This can effectively decrease P_aco_2 to normal values, as the CO_2 dissociation curve is linear within the physiologic range. However, this increase in ventilation cannot adequately increase arterial O_2 (P_aO_2), due to the plateauing of the oxygen–hemoglobin dissociation curve in the upper working range of Pao_2 values in high V/Q regions.[4]

METABOLIC CARBON DIOXIDE PRODUCTION

Increased $V'CO_2$ is rarely a cause of hypercapnia by itself, as an increased CO_2 load stimulates chemoreceptors, altering $V'e$ accordingly. Nonetheless, in patients who cannot mount a sufficient increase in $V'e$, such as in neuromuscular disease, increased $V'CO_2$ (for instance as occurs in hyperthermia, thyrotoxicosis, resistive breathing, or exercise) may contribute to elevating P_aco_2.[5]

The respiratory quotient, R, is the ratio of $V'CO_2$ to oxygen consumption ($V'O_2$): $V'CO_2/V'O_2$. As the stoichiometry of aerobic respiration is altered by food source, altering food types may influence $V'CO_2$. For instance, a diet of pure carbohydrate (CHO) will produce a greater amount of CO_2 per mole of CHO ($R = 1$ for glucose) than a diet of pure fat ($R = 0.7$ for palmitic acid).[6] Such a diet can lead to respiratory distress secondary to excessive CO_2 loads.[7]

DEFENDING AGAINST HYPERCAPNIA AND THE VULNERABILITIES OF RESPIRATION IN SLEEP

Protecting against the development of chronic hypercapnia relies on maintaining adequate ventilation, which can only occur if the capacity of the respiratory system (muscles and control center) matches the load ($V'CO_2$, elastic load, and resistive load). Disorders that impair central drive, neuromuscular transmission to the respiratory muscles, respiratory muscle structure and function, and/or chest wall and lung mechanics may lead to the development of hypercapnia (**Fig. 2**).

ANATOMY AND PHYSIOLOGY OF VENTILATORY CONTROL

The pre-Bötzinger complex (PBC), located within the ventrolateral medulla, is the central region involved in inspiratory pattern generation.[8,9] Axons from the PBC project to breathing-related brainstem premotor regions, which connect with motor neurons driving respiratory pump muscles and maintaining airway patency.[10,11] In the postinspiration phase, controlled by a group of neurons medial to the nucleus of cranial nerve VII, contraction of laryngeal adductor muscles occurs simultaneous to length contraction of the diaphragm, thus hindering lung deflation to assist alveolar gas

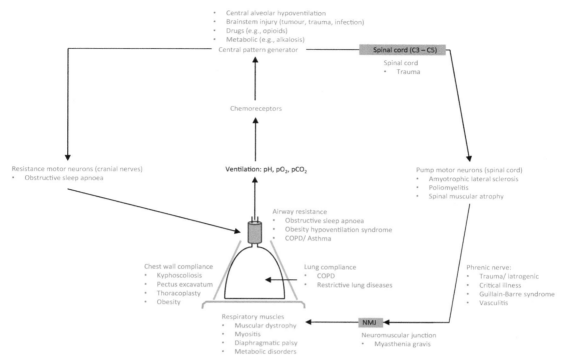

Fig. 2. Anatomic localization of diseases leading to hypoventilation.

exchange.[12] Active expiration is governed by the retrotrapezoid nucleus (RTN)/parafacial respiratory group,[13] driving expiratory muscles, including the abdominal and internal intercostal muscles. Hypercapnia disinhibits these groups to promote active expiration.[14] The hypothalamus and pons are other areas involved in the maintenance and fine tuning of ventilation.[15]

Key to maintaining steady state levels of Pao_2, $Paco_2$, and pH is chemoreception, in concert with feedback provided by mechanoreceptors, irritant receptors, and basal metabolic rate. The central chemoreceptors are situated within several locations in the lower brainstem, the most prominent being the RTN.[16,17] These glutamatergic neurons on the ventral surface of the medulla rely on the expression of the transcription factor paired-like homeobox 2B (PHOX2B) for neuronal development.[18] Mutations in PHOX2B are responsible for the congenital central hypoventilation syndrome.[15] It is estimated that approximately two-thirds of the ventilatory response to $Paco_2$/pH is modulated via the central chemoreceptor, and the response is linear.[19]

The peripheral chemoreceptors are predominantly located within the carotid body.[20] While they are also sensitive to changes in pH and $Paco_2$,[21] their predominant role is to sense arterial hypoxemia.[22] Other regions—including the medulla, kidneys, and spinal cord—also sense O_2

and modulate the hypoxic ventilatory response.[22] The response to hypoxia is curvilinear, such that $V'e$ increases significantly once Pao_2 falls below 60 mm Hg.[23]

SLEEP STATE-RELATED VULNERABILITIES

Sleep onset is accompanied by a reduction in motor output to upper airway resistance muscles, intercostal muscles, and the diaphragm. This decreases upper airway muscle activity, thereby increasing upper airway compliance and reducing upper airway luminal diameter.[24–26] Furthermore, the neurocompensatory pharyngeal reflex for increased mechanical loads is lost due to the loss of the wakefulness drive to breathe.[27] This decoupling of load-compensation results in a reduction in minute ventilation of 6% to 7% during nonrapid eye movement sleep and 10% to 15% during rapid eye movement (REM) sleep,[28] further accentuated by reduced hypoxic and hypercapnic ventilatory responsiveness.[29] In addition, tonic activity to the tongue, pharyngeal, laryngeal, and intercostal muscles also diminish during REM, whereby the maintenance of ventilation is entirely dependent on the diaphragm and is vulnerable to upper airway narrowing and closure.[30,31] Despite these circumstances, the net result in normal adults is a clinically insignificant rise in $Paco_2$ during sleep, partly the consequence of a lowered metabolic rate reducing O_2 consumption, thus reducing CO_2 production, in sleep.[32]

Sleep is also accompanied by a reduction in the functional residual capacity (FRC), the resting state of the respiratory system where inward elastic recoil of the lung is balanced by the outward recoil of the chest wall.[33] This is postulated to result from an increased thoracic blood volume (decreasing lung compliance) and relative diaphragm hypotonia, coupled with the change in static respiratory mechanics that occurs in the supine position.[34]

THE MECHANISM OF OXYGEN-INDUCED HYPERCAPNIA

First recognized in the 1930s, O_2-induced hypercapnia is an important pathologic consequence of uncontrolled O_2 therapy in neuromuscular disease, obesity hypoventilation syndrome (OHS), chronic obstructive pulmonary disease (COPD), severe asthma, and community-acquired pneumonia.[35] Multiple mechanisms are thought to contribute, summarised below and in **Fig. 3**.

As chronic hypercapnia develops in patients with CHRF, the compensatory metabolic alkalosis that ensues increases the buffering capacity of the cerebrospinal fluid (CSF),[36,37] such that hypercapnia-induced CSF acidosis does not occur. This results in a reduced ventilatory response to CO_2,[38] leading to the hypoxic drive to breathe becoming an important stimulus for ventilation.[39] Though initially considered the main mechanism for O_2-induced hypercapnia in COPD, the fall in respiratory drive and $V'e$ that occurs in patients with COPD subject to high fractions of O_2 is insufficient to explain the magnitude of rise in Pa_{CO_2}.[40,41]

The mechanism now regarded as the predominant factor in O_2-induced hypercapnia in COPD is increased Vd/Vt.[42] Increased O_2 administration reduces hypoxic pulmonary vasoconstriction,[43] thereby increasing perfusion to poorly ventilated lung regions and increasing Vd/Vt.[44] The Vd/Vt is further increased by the mechanism of absorption atelectasis, whereby high concentrations of O_2 facilitate atelectasis in low V/Q units where the pulmonary capillary uptake of O_2 exceeds the rate of fresh supply of O_2 via alveolar ventilation.[45]

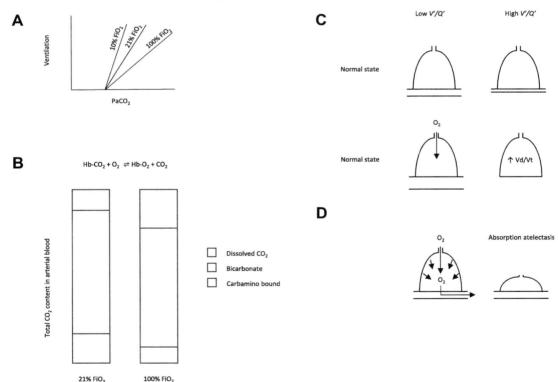

Fig. 3. (*A*) Oxygen-induced blunting of hypercapnic ventilatory response. (*B*) Haldane effect: Oxyhemoglobin (Hb-O_2) has reduced affinity for carbamino-bound hemoglobin (Hb-CO_2) such that increased Hb-O_2 increases the amount of dissolved CO_2. (*C*) Increased Vd/Vt: Hyperoxia reduces hypoxic pulmonary vasoconstriction, such that perfusion is "stolen" from high V/Q units, thereby increasing Vd/Vt. (*D*) Absorption atelectasis: Supplemental O_2 displaces nitrogen. When the rate of pulmonary capillary O_2 uptake exceeds supply of O_2 via ventilation in low V/Q units, alveoli collapse, contributing to impaired CO_2 clearance.

The Haldane effect is the third (and least prominent) mechanism of O_2-induced hypercapnia.[46] This refers to the decreased affinity of oxyhemoglobin for CO_2, such that for a given CO_2 blood content, increased oxygenation leads to increases in Pa_{CO_2}[47] (see **Fig. 3**).

CENTRAL DISORDERS ASSOCIATED WITH HYPOVENTILATION

The central respiratory rhythm generator lies within the medulla. Congenital central hypoventilation syndrome is characterized by sleep-related hypoventilation and the presence of a PHOX2B mutation, related to an autosomal dominant polyalanine repeat expansion.[48] In this syndrome, the hypercapnic ventilatory response is attenuated, particularly during sleep,[49] most likely due to failed central integration of chemoreceptor input.[50]

Rapid onset obesity, hypoventilation, hypothalamic dysfunction, and autonomic dysregulation syndrome is another such disorder. Aside from the many manifestations of hypothalamic dysfunction characteristic of this disorder, central apnea, obstructive sleep apnea (OSA), and abnormal hypercapnic ventilatory responsiveness occur, leading to diurnal hypercapnia.[51] While the pathophysiology of this condition remains poorly understood,[52] accumulating evidence suggest a paraneoplastic or autoimmune mechanism.[53]

NEUROMUSCULAR DISEASES AND THE MECHANISMS PROMOTING CHRONIC HYPERCAPNIA

While several different neuromuscular diseases can lead to CHRF, the common endpoint is respiratory muscle weakness, leading to load-compensation failure. Not uncommonly, the first presentation of a neuromuscular disease is awake hypercapnic respiratory failure.[54]

Inspiratory muscle weakness, predominantly affecting the diaphragm, contributes to reduced contractile function and respiratory muscle fatigue,[55] resulting in a reflexive rapid shallow breathing pattern to minimize the energy cost of breathing.[56] This further contributes to increased Vd/Vt, and thus chronic hypercapnia. This pattern of breathing may also contribute to reduced compliance and increased elastic loading.[57,58] Expiratory muscle weakness usually accompanies inspiratory muscle weakness, leading to an impaired cough and swallow reflex, contributing to retained secretions, atelectasis, and aspiration risk.[59]

To compensate for reduced force-generating capacity, central drive to respiratory muscle motor neurons is often augmented.[60] While studies in patients with neuromuscular disease have highlighted a reduction in hypercapnic ventilatory responsiveness, suggesting a reduced chemical drive to breathe,[61,62] assessing such responses is difficult due to the reduced force-generating capacity of the respiratory muscles. In contrast, direct diaphragmatic electromyography measurements in the face of increasing CO_2 levels showed similar augmentation in activity in controls compared to patients with neuromuscular disease.[62] It is believed that chronic hypoventilation, through the mechanism of bicarbonate retention (and consequent CSF alkalosis), more likely leads to reduced hypercapnic ventilatory responsiveness. Nocturnal noninvasive ventilatory support (NIV) significantly improved the mean hypercapnic ventilatory response in a group of patients with hypercapnia, the majority of whom had neuromuscular disease, with strong correlation to changes in awake Pa_{CO_2}.[63]

Nocturnal hypoventilation is an early predictor of awake hypercapnia in patients with neuromuscular disease.[64] Initially, repetitive desaturation events occur during phasic REM sleep, related to REM muscle atonia of the intercostal muscles and reliance on a weakened diaphragm. The raised CO_2 triggers frequent arousals from sleep, suppressing REM sleep and causing sleep fragmentation.[65,66] Furthermore, sleep deprivation may contribute to hypoventilation by blunting hypercapnic ventilatory responsiveness[67] and reducing arousal responses to hypercapnia.[68]

RESTRICTIVE CHEST WALL DISORDERS AND THE MECHANISMS PROMOTING CHRONIC HYPERCAPNIA

The restrictive chest wall disorders are a group of conditions with the common pathophysiology of decreased chest wall compliance. They include conditions such as kyphoscoliosis, thoracoplasty, and pectus excavatum. Respiratory impairment occurs due to distortion of the thorax, leading to reduced respiratory system compliance (C_{RS}), primarily due to reduced chest wall compliance.[69] Lung compliance can also be reduced because of reduced lung volumes and microatelectasis.[70]

Accompanying reduced C_{RS}, work of breathing increases, and patients develop a rapid shallow breathing pattern, leading to increased Vd/Vt.[71] Airway resistance may also increase due to retained secretions, chronic inflammation, comorbid asthma/COPD or even distortion of the large airways.[72] Microatelectasis and reduced lung volumes impair V/Q matching,[73] while inspiratory muscle strength may be reduced due to abnormal chest wall geometry causing muscle inefficiency,[74] and later from the effects of hypercapnia.[75] The hypercapnic ventilatory response is also reduced in individuals with awake hypercapnic failure.[76] The most common abnormality during sleep is REM hypoventilation, which occurs due to reliance on the diaphragm to maintain ventilation.[77] Notably, the hypercapnic ventilatory response improves after initiation of NIV.[63]

OBESITY HYPOVENTILATION SYNDROME AND THE MECHANISMS PROMOTING HYPERCAPNIA

OHS is the presence of awake hypoventilation (Pa_{CO_2} >45 mm Hg) in an obese individual without any other identified cause of daytime hypercapnia.[78] Like most disorders associated with CHRF, the mechanisms leading to awake hypercapnia in OHS are multifactorial.

The most important physiologic derangement is sleep-disordered breathing. Most patients with OHS have concurrent OSA,[79] related to excessive upper airway fat deposition, lower lung volumes, and increased upper airway collapsibility.[80] Rostral fluid shifts also cause increases in critical closing pressure due to upper airway congestion.[81] Pure sleep-related hypoventilation occurs less commonly, affecting approximately 10% of patients.[82] Awake hypercapnia is believed to develop due to decreased CO_2 clearance between apneic events,[83,84] promoting bicarbonate retention, and blunting the hypercapnic ventilatory response.[36] Treatment of sleep-disordered breathing improves awake hypercapnia.[82]

Abnormalities in pulmonary mechanics and gas exchange also develop. Excess chest wall and abdominal adipose tissue contribute to reducing C_{RS},[85] decreasing the FRC and significantly reducing the expiratory reserve volume (ERV).[86,87] Airway resistance also increases due to reductions in airway caliber at lower resting lung volumes.[88] Associated with the reduction in ERV, premature closure of small airways occurs, contributing to V/Q mismatching, basal atelectasis, and the development of intrinsic positive end-expiratory pressure.[89] This leads to an increased inspiratory threshold loading, especially in the supine position,[90] and work of breathing increases.[91,92] To compensate, patients adopt a shallow breathing pattern, further contributing to increased Vd/Vt.[93]

Evidence indicates that respiratory muscles are impaired in OHS. Maximum inspiratory strength is reduced in comparison to obese individuals with eucapnia.[94] Respiratory muscle endurance is also reduced in patients with OHS, while patients with OHS who used NIV had improved respiratory muscle endurance in comparison to nonusers, perhaps due to resting of chronically fatigued muscles during sleep.[95,96] Lipid accumulation within the diaphragm may also occur. In mice models, this leads to lipotoxicity-induced diaphragm dysfunction.[97]

While eucapnic obese individuals augment their neural respiratory drive compared to normal weight healthy individuals to counter the increased load on the respiratory system,[98] patients with OHS lack this compensatory response,[99] demonstrating reduced hypoxic[100] and hypercapnic ventilatory responsiveness.[101] This is believed to occur due to impaired CO_2 clearance at night secondary to sleep-disordered breathing, causing bicarbonate retention. Supporting this mechanism, treatment with NIV has been shown to improve neural respiratory drive in patients with OHS.[102]

Another possible factor reducing respiratory drive is leptin resistance. Leptin, an adipokine protein encoded by the human obese (ob) gene, is produced by adipocytes. Its role is pleiotropic, having appetite-suppressing effects, increasing metabolic rate, increasing respiratory drive, and maintaining upper airway patency.[103–106] Elevated leptin levels are found in patients with OHS and could be related to leptin resistance.[107,108] Studies in mice have shown consistent results. For instance, ob/ob mice (deficient in leptin) hypoventilate in sleep, and this effect was able to be attenuated by leptin administration, with improved chemoresponsiveness to CO_2.[105,109] Additionally, focal application of leptin to hypoglossal motor neurons in a leptin-resistant mice model of obesity led to improved upper airway patency.[110] Whether CNS leptin administration may reverse reduced neural respiratory drive in humans is yet to be determined.

Overproduction of CO_2 appears to be another factor contributing to diurnal hypercapnia. Patients with OHS who had OSA of similar severity to controls with eucapnia had higher CO_2 production ($V'CO_2$), with similar indices of alveolar ventilation.[111] A recent study highlighted the potential for dietary modification to reduce $V'CO_2$ by using a ketogenic diet enriched in dietary fat to reduce R, thereby reducing awake Pa_{CO_2}.[112,113] However, this effect may have been partly mediated by ketone body–associated metabolic acidosis, loop gain stabilizing effects, and acute weight loss.[112]

CHRONIC OBSTRUCTIVE PULMONARY DISEASE AND THE MECHANISMS PRODUCING HYPERCAPNIA

While hypercapnia in COPD is commonly linked to the severity of airflow obstruction, it can also develop in patients with milder airflow obstruction, and in patients with comorbid OSA.[114,115]

Multiple mechanisms contribute to an imbalance in the load–capacity–drive relationship that eventually leads to chronic hypercapnia in COPD.

Airflow obstruction, the hallmark of COPD, develops through chronic inflammation in small airways,[116] while accompanying alveolar damage causes a reduction in elastic recoil and surface area for gas exchange.[117] Static hyperinflation develops, with a larger FRC producing greater inward elastic recoil pressure to counterbalance outward chest wall recoil pressure.[118] With disease progression, end-expiratory lung volume increases, eventually moving above the relaxation volume of the chest wall. The mechanical time constant for lung emptying then increases, resulting in gas trapping at end-expiration,[119] creating increased threshold inspiratory loading. As the FRC increases toward total lung capacity, the inspiratory reserve volume decreases and Vt falls. In conjunction with altered V/Q, both Vd/Vt and ventilatory inefficiency increase,[120] while hyperinflation alters the geometry of the diaphragm, imposing further mechanical constraint.[121]

Nocturnal hypoventilation also occurs frequently in patients with COPD, as the reduced ventilatory drive during sleep is unable to compensate for the mechanical load imposed by increased airway resistance and hyperinflation, becoming particularly severe during REM sleep.[77,122] This too may contribute to awake hypercapnia.[123]

SUMMARY

CHRF is a common clinical problem and an endpoint in many diseases that affect the load–capacity–drive balance. Ultimately, the underlying pathophysiology relates to alveolar hypoventilation that can be explained in turn by multiple mechanisms that act to increase metabolic CO_2 production, decrease minute ventilation, and/or increase Vd/Vt. Sleep-related hypoventilation is believed to play a central role and is often the first abnormality detected prior to the development of diurnal hypercapnia.

CLINICS CARE POINTS

- CHRF is a common problem encountered in sleep and respiratory clinics.
- The underlying mechanism is alveolar hypoventilation, which occurs because of load (elastic, resistive, and metabolic), capacity (respiratory pump efficiency), and drive (neural respiratory drive) imbalance.

- Elevated $Paco_2$ can occur through multiple mechanisms that (1) increase metabolic CO_2 production (rarely the only reason), (2) reduce minute ventilation, and/or (3) increase Vd/Vt.
- Because sleep-related hypoventilation may be an early sign of diurnal hypercapnia, timely assessment of nocturnal gas-exchange with polysomnography/oxycapnography is recommended in patients where sleep-related hypoventilation is suspected.

DISCLOSURE

The authors have nothing to disclose.

REFERENCES

1. Wiklund L. Carbon dioxide formation and elimination in man. Recent theories and possible consequences. Ups J Med Sci 1996;101(1):35–67.
2. Krebs HA, Johnson WA. The role of citric acid in intermediate metabolism in animal tissues. FEBS Lett 1980;117(Suppl):K1–10.
3. Roussos C. The failing ventilatory pump. Lung 1982;160(2):59–84.
4. West JB. Causes of and compensations for hypoxemia and hypercapnia. Compr Physiol 2011;1(3): 1541–53.
5. Weinberger SE, Schwartzstein RM, Weiss JW. Hypercapnia. N Engl J Med 1989;321(18):1223–31.
6. Askanazi J, Nordenstrom J, Rosenbaum SH, et al. Nutrition for the patient with respiratory failure: glucose vs. fat. Anesthesiology 1981;54(5):373–7.
7. Covelli HD, Black JW, Olsen MS, et al. Respiratory failure precipitated by high carbohydrate loads. Ann Intern Med 1981;95(5):579–81.
8. Smith JC, Ellenberger HH, Ballanyi K, et al. Pre-Botzinger complex: a brainstem region that may generate respiratory rhythm in mammals. Science 1991;254(5032):726–9.
9. Schwarzacher SW, Rub U, Deller T. Neuroanatomical characteristics of the human pre-Botzinger complex and its involvement in neurodegenerative brainstem diseases. Brain 2011;134(Pt 1):24–35.
10. Smith JC, Morrison DE, Ellenberger HH, et al. Brainstem projections to the major respiratory neuron populations in the medulla of the cat. J Comp Neurol 1989;281(1):69–96.
11. Tan W, Pagliardini S, Yang P, et al. Projections of preBotzinger complex neurons in adult rats. J Comp Neurol 2010;518(10):1862–78.
12. Dutschmann M, Jones SE, Subramanian HH, et al. The physiological significance of postinspiration in respiratory control. Prog Brain Res 2014;212: 113–30.

13. Feldman JL, Mitchell GS, Nattie EE. Breathing: rhythmicity, plasticity, chemosensitivity. Annu Rev Neurosci 2003;26:239–66.

14. de Britto AA, Moraes DJ. Non-chemosensitive parafacial neurons simultaneously regulate active expiration and airway patency under hypercapnia in rats. J Physiol 2017;595(6):2043–64.

15. Baughn JM, Matarese CA. Control of breathing and central hypoventilation syndromes. Sleep Med Clin 2023;18(2):161–71.

16. Chowdhuri S, Badr MS. Control of ventilation in health and disease. Chest 2017;151(4):917–29.

17. SheikhBahaei S, Marina N, Rajani V, et al. Contributions of carotid bodies, retrotrapezoid nucleus neurons and preBotzinger complex astrocytes to the CO(2) -sensitive drive for breathing. J Physiol 2024;602(1):223–40.

18. Feldman JL, Del Negro CA, Gray PA. Understanding the rhythm of breathing: so near, yet so far. Annu Rev Physiol 2013;75:423–52.

19. Forster HV, Smith CA. Contributions of central and peripheral chemoreceptors to the ventilatory response to CO2/H+. J Appl Physiol 2010;108(4):989–94.

20. de Castro F. Towards the sensory nature of the carotid body: hering, de castro and heymansdagger. Front Neuroanat 2009;3:23.

21. Lahiri S, Forster RE 2nd. CO2/H(+) sensing: peripheral and central chemoreception. Int J Biochem Cell Biol 2003;35(10):1413–35.

22. Dempsey JA, Gibbons TD. Rethinking O(2) , CO(2) and breathing during wakefulness and sleep. J Physiol 2023. https://doi.org/10.1113/JP284551.

23. Prabhakar NR, Peng YJ. Peripheral chemoreceptors in health and disease. J Appl Physiol 2004;96(1):359–66.

24. Mezzanotte WS, Tangel DJ, White DP. Influence of sleep onset on upper-airway muscle activity in apnea patients versus normal controls. Am J Respir Crit Care Med 1996;153(6 Pt 1):1880–7.

25. Fogel RB, Trinder J, White DP, et al. The effect of sleep onset on upper airway muscle activity in patients with sleep apnoea versus controls. J Physiol 2005;564(Pt 2):549–62.

26. Tangel DJ, Mezzanotte WS, White DP. Influence of sleep on tensor palatini EMG and upper airway resistance in normal men. J Appl Physiol 1991;70(6):2574–81.

27. Gugger M, Molloy J, Gould GA, et al. Ventilatory and arousal responses to added inspiratory resistance during sleep. Am Rev Respir Dis 1989;140(5):1301–7.

28. Douglas NJ, White DP, Pickett CK, et al. Respiration during sleep in normal man. Thorax 1982;37(11):840–4.

29. Berthon-Jones M, Sullivan CE. Ventilation and arousal responses to hypercapnia in normal sleeping humans. J Appl Physiol Respir Environ Exerc Physiol 1984;57(1):59–67.

30. Tabachnik E, Muller NL, Bryan AC, et al. Changes in ventilation and chest wall mechanics during sleep in normal adolescents. J Appl Physiol Respir Environ Exerc Physiol 1981;51(3):557–64.

31. McSharry DG, Saboisky JP, Deyoung P, et al. Physiological mechanisms of upper airway hypotonia during REM sleep. Sleep 2014;37(3):561–9.

32. White DP, Weil JV, Zwillich CW. Metabolic rate and breathing during sleep. J Appl Physiol 1985;59(2):384–91.

33. Hudgel DW, Devadatta P. Decrease in functional residual capacity during sleep in normal humans. J Appl Physiol Respir Environ Exerc Physiol 1984;57(5):1319–22.

34. Casey KR, Cantillo KO, Brown LK. Sleep-related hypoventilation/hypoxemic syndromes. Chest 2007;131(6):1936–48.

35. Sarkar M, Madabhavi I, Kadakol N. Oxygen-induced hypercapnia: physiological mechanisms and clinical implications. Monaldi Arch Chest Dis 2022;93(3).

36. Goldring RM, Turino GM, Heinemann HO. Respiratory-renal adjustments in chronic hypercapnia in man. Extracellular bicarbonate concentration and the regulation of ventilation. Am J Med 1971;51(6):772–84.

37. Warner DS, Turner DM, Kassell NF. Time-dependent effects of prolonged hypercapnia on cerebrovascular parameters in dogs: acid-base chemistry. Stroke 1987;18(1):142–9.

38. Oppersma E, Doorduin J, van der Hoeven JG, et al. The effect of metabolic alkalosis on the ventilatory response in healthy subjects. Respir Physiol Neurobiol 2018;249:47–53.

39. Campbell EJ. Respiratory failure: the relation between oxygen concentrations of inspired air and arterial blood. Lancet 1960;2(7140):10–1.

40. Aubier M, Murciano D, Fournier M, et al. Central respiratory drive in acute respiratory failure of patients with chronic obstructive pulmonary disease. Am Rev Respir Dis 1980;122(2):191–9.

41. Aubier M, Murciano D, Milic-Emili J, et al. Effects of the administration of O2 on ventilation and blood gases in patients with chronic obstructive pulmonary disease during acute respiratory failure. Am Rev Respir Dis 1980;122(5):747–54.

42. Sassoon CS, Hassell KT, Mahutte CK. Hyperoxic-induced hypercapnia in stable chronic obstructive pulmonary disease. Am Rev Respir Dis 1987;135(4):907–11.

43. Slingo ME. Oxygen-sensing pathways and the pulmonary circulation. J Physiol 2023. https://doi.org/10.1113/JP284591.

44. Robertson HT. Dead space: the physiology of wasted ventilation. Eur Respir J 2015;45(6):1704–16.

45. Dantzker DR, Wagner PD, West JB. Proceedings: instability of poorly ventilated lung units during oxygen breathing. J Physiol 1974;242(2):72P.

46. Christiansen J, Douglas CG, Haldane JS. The absorption and dissociation of carbon dioxide by human blood. J Physiol 1914;48(4):244–71.

47. Lenfant C. Arterial-alveolar difference in PCO2 during air and oxygen breathing. J Appl Physiol 1966; 21(4):1356–62.

48. Maloney MA, Kun SS, Keens TG, et al. Congenital central hypoventilation syndrome: diagnosis and management. Expet Rev Respir Med 2018;12(4): 283–92.

49. Fu C, Xue J, Wang R, et al. Chemosensitive Phox2b-expressing neurons are crucial for hypercapnic ventilatory response in the nucleus tractus solitarius. J Physiol 2017;595(14):4973–89.

50. Marcus CL, Bautista DB, Amihyia A, et al. Hypercapneic arousal responses in children with congenital central hypoventilation syndrome. Pediatrics 1991;88(5):993–8.

51. Lazea C, Sur L, Florea M. ROHHAD (Rapid-onset obesity with hypoventilation, hypothalamic dysfunction, autonomic dysregulation) syndromewhat every pediatrician should know about the etiopathogenesis, diagnosis and treatment: a review. Int J Gen Med 2021;14:319–26.

52. Khaytin I, Victor AK, Barclay SF, et al. Rapid-onset obesity with hypothalamic dysfunction, hypoventilation, and autonomic dysregulation (ROHHAD): a collaborative review of the current understanding. Clin Auton Res 2023;33(3):251–68.

53. Mandel-Brehm C, Benson LA, Tran B, et al. ZSCAN1 autoantibodies are associated with pediatric paraneoplastic ROHHAD. Ann Neurol 2022; 92(2):279–91.

54. Keunen RW, Lambregts PC, Op de Coul AA, et al. Respiratory failure as initial symptom of acid maltase deficiency. J Neurol Neurosurg Psychiatry 1984;47(5):549–52.

55. Roussos C, Zakynthinos S. Fatigue of the respiratory muscles. Intensive Care Med 1996;22(2): 134–55.

56. Misuri G, Lanini B, Gigliotti F, et al. Mechanism of CO(2) retention in patients with neuromuscular disease. Chest 2000;117(2):447–53.

57. Estenne M, Gevenois PA, Kinnear W, et al. Lung volume restriction in patients with chronic respiratory muscle weakness: the role of microatelectasis. Thorax 1993;48(7):698–701.

58. De Troyer A, Borenstein S, Cordier R. Analysis of lung volume restriction in patients with respiratory muscle weakness. Thorax 1980;35(8): 603–10.

59. Ambrosino N, Carpene N, Gherardi M. Chronic respiratory care for neuromuscular diseases in adults. Eur Respir J 2009;34(2):444–51.

60. Baydur A. Respiratory muscle strength and control of ventilation in patients with neuromuscular disease. Chest 1991;99(2):330–8.

61. Begin R, Bureau MA, Lupien L, et al. Control and modulation of respiration in Steinert's myotonic dystrophy. Am Rev Respir Dis 1980;121(2):281–9.

62. Gigliotti F, Pizzi A, Duranti R, et al. Control of breathing in patients with limb girdle dystrophy: a controlled study. Thorax 1995;50(9):962–8.

63. Nickol AH, Hart N, Hopkinson NS, et al. Mechanisms of improvement of respiratory failure in patients with restrictive thoracic disease treated with non-invasive ventilation. Thorax 2005;60(9):754–60.

64. Piper A. Sleep abnormalities associated with neuromuscular disease: pathophysiology and evaluation. Semin Respir Crit Care Med 2002;23(3): 211–9.

65. Arnulf I, Similowski T, Salachas F, et al. Sleep disorders and diaphragmatic function in patients with amyotrophic lateral sclerosis. Am J Respir Crit Care Med 2000;161(3 Pt 1):849–56.

66. White JE, Drinnan MJ, Smithson AJ, et al. Respiratory muscle activity and oxygenation during sleep in patients with muscle weakness. Eur Respir J 1995;8(5):807–14.

67. White DP, Douglas NJ, Pickett CK, et al. Sleep deprivation and the control of ventilation. Am Rev Respir Dis 1983;128(6):984–6.

68. Li Y, Panossian LA, Zhang J, et al. Effects of chronic sleep fragmentation on wake-active neurons and the hypercapnic arousal response. Sleep 2014;37(1):51–64.

69. Baydur A, Swank SM, Stiles CM, et al. Respiratory mechanics in anesthetized young patients with kyphoscoliosis. Immediate and delayed effects of corrective spinal surgery. Chest 1990;97(5): 1157–64.

70. Bergofsky EH. Respiratory failure in disorders of the thoracic cage. Am Rev Respir Dis 1979; 119(4):643–69.

71. Tzelepis GE. Chest wall diseases: respiratory pathophysiology. Clin Chest Med 2018;39(2):281–96.

72. van Noord JA, Cauberghs M, Van de Woestijne KP, et al. Total respiratory resistance and reactance in ankylosing spondylitis and kyphoscoliosis. Eur Respir J 1991;4(8):945–51.

73. Secker-Walker RH, Ho JE, Gill IS. Observations on regional ventilation and perfusion in kyphoscoliosis. Respiration 1979;38(4):194–203.

74. Roussos C, Macklem PT. The respiratory muscles. N Engl J Med 1982;307(13):786–97.

75. Juan G, Calverley P, Talamo C, et al. Effect of carbon dioxide on diaphragmatic function in human beings. N Engl J Med 1984;310(14):874–9.

76. Bergofsky EH, Turino GM, Fishman AP. Cardiorespiratory failure in kyphoscoliosis. Medicine (Baltim) 1959;38:263–317.

77. Piper AJ, Yee BJ. Hypoventilation syndromes. Compr Physiol 2014;4(4):1639–76.

78. Randerath W, Verbraecken J, Andreas S, et al. Definition, discrimination, diagnosis and treatment of central breathing disturbances during sleep. Eur Respir J 2017;49(1):1600959.

79. Berger KI, Ayappa I, Chatr-Amontri B, et al. Obesity hypoventilation syndrome as a spectrum of respiratory disturbances during sleep. Chest 2001;120(4):1231–8.

80. Levy P, Kohler M, McNicholas WT, et al. Obstructive sleep apnoea syndrome. Nat Rev Dis Prim 2015;1:15015.

81. White LH, Bradley TD. Role of nocturnal rostral fluid shift in the pathogenesis of obstructive and central sleep apnoea. J Physiol 2013;591(5): 1179–93.

82. Masa JF, Pepin JL, Borel JC, et al. Obesity hypoventilation syndrome. Eur Respir Rev 2019; 28(151):180097.

83. Berger KI, Ayappa I, Sorkin IB, et al. CO(2) homeostasis during periodic breathing in obstructive sleep apnea. J Appl Physiol 2000;88(1):257–64.

84. Berger KI, Ayappa I, Sorkin IB, et al. Postevent ventilation as a function of CO(2) load during respiratory events in obstructive sleep apnea. J Appl Physiol 2002;93(3):917–24.

85. Pelosi P, Croci M, Ravagnan I, et al. Total respiratory system, lung, and chest wall mechanics in sedated-paralyzed postoperative morbidly obese patients. Chest 1996;109(1):144–51.

86. Hodgson LE, Murphy PB, Hart N. Respiratory management of the obese patient undergoing surgery. J Thorac Dis 2015;7(5):943–52.

87. Piper AJ, Grunstein RR. Big breathing: the complex interaction of obesity, hypoventilation, weight loss, and respiratory function. J Appl Physiol 2010; 108(1):199–205.

88. Zerah F, Harf A, Perlemuter L, et al. Effects of obesity on respiratory resistance. Chest 1993; 103(5):1470–6.

89. Pankow W, Podszus T, Gutheil T, et al. Expiratory flow limitation and intrinsic positive end-expiratory pressure in obesity. J Appl Physiol 1998;85(4): 1236–43.

90. Mughal MM, Culver DA, Minai OA, et al. Auto-positive end-expiratory pressure: mechanisms and treatment. Cleve Clin J Med 2005;72(9):801–9.

91. Lin CK, Lin CC. Work of breathing and respiratory drive in obesity. Respirology 2012;17(3):402–11.

92. Lee MY, Lin CC, Shen SY, et al. Work of breathing in eucapnic and hypercapnic sleep apnea syndrome. Respiration 2009;77(2):146–53.

93. Chlif M, Keochkerian D, Choquet D, et al. Effects of obesity on breathing pattern, ventilatory neural drive and mechanics. Respir Physiol Neurobiol 2009;168(3):198–202.

94. Sharp JT, Druz WS, Kondragunta VR. Diaphragmatic responses to body position changes in obese patients with obstructive sleep apnea. Am Rev Respir Dis 1986;133(1):32–7.

95. Ambrosino N, Montagna T, Nava S, et al. Short term effect of intermittent negative pressure ventilation in COPD patients with respiratory failure. Eur Respir J 1990;3(5):502–8.

96. Dusgun ES, Aslan GK, Abanoz ES, et al. Respiratory muscle endurance in obesity hypoventilation syndrome. Respir Care 2022;67(5):526–33.

97. Xiang X, Zhu Y, Pan X, et al. ER stress aggravates diaphragm weakness through activating PERK/JNK signaling in obesity hypoventilation syndrome. Obesity 2023;31(8):2076–89.

98. Steier J, Jolley CJ, Seymour J, et al. Neural respiratory drive in obesity. Thorax 2009;64(8):719–25.

99. Lopata M, Onal E. Mass loading, sleep apnea, and the pathogenesis of obesity hypoventilation. Am Rev Respir Dis 1982;126(4):640–5.

100. Zwillich CW, Sutton FD, Pierson DJ, et al. Decreased hypoxic ventilatory drive in the obesity-hypoventilation syndrome. Am J Med 1975;59(3):343–8.

101. Verbraecken J, McNicholas WT. Respiratory mechanics and ventilatory control in overlap syndrome and obesity hypoventilation. Respir Res 2013;14(1):132.

102. Onofri A, Patout M, Kaltsakas G, et al. Neural respiratory drive and cardiac function in patients with obesity hypoventilation syndrome following initiation of non-invasive ventilation. J Thorac Dis 2018;10(Suppl 1):S135–43.

103. Kelesidis T, Kelesidis I, Chou S, et al. Narrative review: the role of leptin in human physiology: emerging clinical applications. Ann Intern Med 2010;152(2):93–100.

104. Bassi M, Furuya WI, Menani JV, et al. Leptin into the ventrolateral medulla facilitates chemorespiratory response in leptin-deficient (ob/ob) mice. Acta Physiol 2014;211(1):240–8.

105. O'Donnell CP, Schaub CD, Haines AS, et al. Leptin prevents respiratory depression in obesity. Am J Respir Crit Care Med 1999;159(5 Pt 1):1477–84.

106. Yao Q, Pho H, Kirkness J, et al. Localizing effects of leptin on upper airway and respiratory control during sleep. Sleep 2016;39(5):1097–106.

107. Phipps PR, Starritt E, Caterson I, et al. Association of serum leptin with hypoventilation in human obesity. Thorax 2002;57(1):75–6.

108. Campo A, Fruhbeck G, Zulueta JJ, et al. Hyperleptinaemia, respiratory drive and hypercapnic response in obese patients. Eur Respir J 2007; 30(2):223–31.

109. Bassi M, Giusti H, Leite CM, et al. Central leptin replacement enhances chemorespiratory responses in leptin-deficient mice independent of

changes in body weight. Pflügers Archiv 2012; 464(2):145–53.

110. Freire C, Pho H, Kim LJ, et al. Intranasal leptin prevents opioid-induced sleep-disordered breathing in obese mice. Am J Respir Cell Mol Biol 2020; 63(4):502–9.

111. Javaheri S, Simbartl LA. Respiratory determinants of diurnal hypercapnia in obesity hypoventilation syndrome. What does weight have to do with it? Ann Am Thorac Soc 2014;11(6):945–50.

112. Osman A, Gu C, Kim DE, et al. Ketogenic diet acutely improves gas exchange and sleep apnoea in obesity hypoventilation syndrome: a non-randomized crossover study. Respirology 2023; 28(8):784–93.

113. Silberman H, Silberman AW. Parenteral nutrition, biochemistry and respiratory gas exchange. JPEN - J Parenter Enter Nutr 1986;10(2):151–4.

114. McNicholas WT, Hansson D, Schiza S, et al. Sleep in chronic respiratory disease: COPD and hypoventilation disorders. Eur Respir Rev 2019; 28(153):190064.

115. Csoma B, Vulpi MR, Dragonieri S, et al. Hypercapnia in COPD: causes, consequences, and therapy. J Clin Med 2022;11(11):3180.

116. Hogg JC, Macklem PT, Thurlbeck WM. Site and nature of airway obstruction in chronic obstructive lung disease. N Engl J Med 1968;278(25):1355–60.

117. Jolley CJ, Moxham J. A physiological model of patient-reported breathlessness during daily activities in COPD. Eur Respir Rev 2009;18(112):66–79.

118. Brusasco V, Martinez F. Chronic obstructive pulmonary disease. Compr Physiol 2014;4(1):1–31.

119. Hyatt RE. Expiratory flow limitation. J Appl Physiol Respir Environ Exerc Physiol 1983;55(1 Pt 1):1–7.

120. Young IH, Bye PT. Gas exchange in disease: asthma, chronic obstructive pulmonary disease, cystic fibrosis, and interstitial lung disease. Compr Physiol 2011;1(2):663–97.

121. Decramer M. Hyperinflation and respiratory muscle interaction. Eur Respir J 1997;10(4):934–41.

122. Luo YM, He BT, Wu YX, et al. Neural respiratory drive and ventilation in patients with chronic obstructive pulmonary disease during sleep. Am J Respir Crit Care Med 2014;190(2):227–9.

123. O'Donoghue FJ, Catcheside PG, Ellis EE, et al. Sleep hypoventilation in hypercapnic chronic obstructive pulmonary disease: prevalence and associated factors. Eur Respir J 2003;21(6): 977–84.

Assessment of Chronic Hypercapnic Respiratory Failure

Xinhang Tu, MB[a], Alfredo Selim, MD, MPH[b], Bernardo Selim, MD[c],*

KEYWORDS

- Hypercapnia • Alveolar hypoventilation • Respiratory failure • Assessment
- Sleep-related disorders • Obesity hypoventilation syndrome • Overlap syndrome
- Neuromuscular disease

KEY POINTS

- Chronic hypercapnic respiratory failure may be encountered during the evaluation of sleep-related breathing disorders at the sleep clinic.
- The signs and symptoms of chronic hypercapnic respiratory failure may be indistinguishable from those of sleep apnea, characterized by sleep disruption and daytime functional impairment.
- A suspected diagnosis of chronic hypercapnic respiratory failure is based on a comprehensive clinical history and a thorough physical examination.
- Initial testing includes arterial blood gas analysis (to confirm the diagnosis), pulmonary function tests, and chest radiographs, followed by selected testing to establish a suspected etiology.

INTRODUCTION

The respiratory system regulates the exchange of oxygen (O_2) and carbon dioxide (CO_2) between the environment and the body to sustain metabolism. Respiratory failure is the condition where the respiratory system is unable to adequately maintain the normal level of these gases in the body. This can result in a decrease in O_2 levels (hypoxemic respiratory failure) and/or an increase in CO_2 levels in blood (hypercapnic respiratory failure). Respiratory failure may be further classified based on chronicity into acute, chronic, or acute on chronic respiratory failure.

Chronic hypercapnic respiratory failure is conventionally defined by an arterial CO_2 tension ($Paco_2$) of greater than 45 mm Hg and increased serum bicarbonate as a result of metabolic compensation. The diagnosis and successful management of this condition primarily depend on taking a comprehensive patient history and conducting a thorough clinical evaluation to determine the underlying etiology. This article provides a detailed review of the evaluation of patients presenting to the sleep clinic with chronic hypercapnic respiratory failure.

THE PHYSIOLOGY OF PULMONARY VENTILATION

The respiratory system can be divided into 2 main components: the "lung," which is responsible for gas exchange (exchange of O_2 and CO_2 between the lung and the bloodstream), and the "pump," which mediates lung ventilation (exchange of gas between the lung and the environment). The pump consists of the thoracic wall, including ribs and respiratory muscles, the respiratory

[a] Division of Pulmonary and Critical Care Medicine, Mayo Clinic Center for Sleep Medicine, Mayo Clinic, 200 First Street Southwest, Rochester, MN 55905, USA; [b] Department of Emergency Medicine, Boston University School of Medicine, Veterans Affairs Medical Center, 1400 VFW Pkwy, West Roxbury, MA 02132, USA; [c] Division of Pulmonary and Critical Care Medicine, Mayo Clinic Alix School of Medicine, Mayo Clinic Center for Sleep Medicine, Mayo Clinic, 200 First Street Southwest, Rochester, Minnesota 55905, USA
* Corresponding author.
E-mail address: Selim.bernardo@mayo.edu

Sleep Med Clin 19 (2024) 391–403
https://doi.org/10.1016/j.jsmc.2024.04.002

controllers in the central nervous system (CNS), and the peripheral nerves that enable communication between the central controllers and the respiratory muscles.

The physiologic range of Pa_{CO_2} is between 35 and 45 mm Hg. In a stable metabolic state, this range is maintained by the respiratory pump, which generates the alveolar ventilation (VA) and is tightly regulated by central respiratory controllers to match metabolic needs. VA refers to the volume of inhaled air per minute that reaches the regions of the lungs where gas exchange occurs (alveoli). Therefore, hypercapnia may arise from alveolar hypoventilation as a result of a reduction in the volume of air inhaled (tidal volume [Vt]) and/or a decrease in the frequency of breaths taken per minute (respiration rate [RR]). If minute ventilation (MV) is defined as the product of Vt × RR, then alveolar hypoventilation may occur due to a reduction in either or both of these respiratory parameters.[1]

During sleep, there is a mild physiologic increase of Pa_{CO_2} by approximately 2 to 6 mm Hg due to a decreased MV of up to 15%. The primary cause of decreased ventilation during sleep is mainly attributed to decreased Vt without a significant change in RR. This decline occurs gradually and is dependent on the stage of sleep, beginning with the transition from awake to non-rapid eye movement (NREM) sleep, then further decreasing upon entering rapid eye movement (REM) sleep.[2,3]

THE PATHOPHYSIOLOGY OF CHRONIC HYPERCAPNIC RESPIRATORY FAILURE

While failure of the "lung" (eg, pneumonia) mainly results in hypoxemic respiratory failure, failure of any component of the respiratory "pump" might lead to alveolar hypoventilation and hypercapnia. There are three leading causes of pump failure: (1) inadequate output of the respiratory controllers in the CNS resulting in a decreased respiratory drive (eg, intake of opioids); (2) altered neural and neuromuscular transmission (eg, amyotrophic lateral sclerosis [ALS]); and (3) chest wall or muscle abnormalities (eg, morbid obesity, kyphoscoliosis, myopathies). Acute and/or chronic hypercapnia may result from the presence of one or more causes of pump failure as enumerated earlier (**Table 1**).

While most cases of chronic hypercapnic respiratory failures are identified by awake hypercapnia, it is also possible for patients to experience hypercapnic respiratory failure confined to sleep. Based on the International Classification of Sleep Disorders Text Revision (ICSD-3-TR), sleep-related hypoventilation disorders encompass a range of sleep pathologies defined by nocturnal alveolar hypoventilation.[4] The American Academy of Sleep Medicine Manual for the Scoring of Sleep and Associated Events has defined sleep-related hypoventilation in adults based on polysomnographic criteria: Pa_{CO_2} (or surrogate such as end-tidal CO_2 [$ETCO_2$] or transcutaneous CO_2 [$TcCO_2$] tension) greater than 55 mm Hg for ≥ 10 minutes or an increase in Pa_{CO_2} (or surrogate) ≥ 10 mm Hg during sleep (in comparison to an awake supine value) to a value greater than 50 mm Hg for ≥ 10 minutes.[5] In certain sleep-related hypoventilation diseases, the abnormal increase in CO_2 may be confined to sleep periods (eg, congenital central alveolar hypoventilation syndrome) or extend into wakefulness (eg, obesity hypoventilation syndrome [OHS]). In addition, patients diagnosed with chronic hypercapnic respiratory failure as a result of chronic pulmonary or neuromuscular diseases (NMDs; "sleep-related hypoventilation due to a medical disorder") may encounter an additional rise above their awake CO_2 levels during sleep.[4] This phenomenon arises from the convergence of 2 factors during sleep: a physiologic decrease in minute ventilation during sleep and unfavorable changes in respiratory mechanics while supine.

INITIAL CLINIC ASSESSMENT OF CHRONIC HYPERCAPNIC RESPIRATORY FAILURE
Signs and Symptoms of Hypoventilation

Patients with slow onset hypercapnia may be asymptomatic or minimally symptomatic. When present, signs and symptoms of hypercapnia may lack specificity and resemble those of more prevalent sleep-related breathing disorders, such as obstructive or central sleep apnea. Symptoms include fatigue, impaired concentration and cognition, daytime sleepiness, sleep fragmentation, and morning headaches. Other signs and symptoms may elevate the suspicion of non-sleep-related medical disorders, such as dyspnea on exertion, wheezing, chronic cough, and sputum production in a patient who smokes, or ineffective cough and bulbar dysfunction in a patient with an NMD. The physical examination may provide clues in the diagnosis, such as signs of wheezing, hyperinflation, and use of accessory muscles in patients with advanced chronic obstructive pulmonary disease (COPD), or focal neurologic deficits in NMD. Elevated body mass index (BMI), particularly class III obesity (morbid obesity) combined with sleep-related complaints and hypoxemia, may raise the possibility of OHS when other more common causes of hypercapnic respiratory failure have been ruled out.[2]

Table 1
Sleep-related hypoventilation disorders

Categories	Disorders	Pathophysiology
Sleep-related Hypoventilation Disorders		
Ventilatory control abnormalities ("won't breathe")	• Congenital central hypoventilation syndrome (CCHS) • Idiopathic central hypoventilation. • Brainstem diseases or other CNS disorders affecting the ventilatory control centers. • Prolonged use of medications (eg, opioids) or substances.	• For CCHS ventilatory control is affected by mutations in the PHOX2B gene. In animal models, PHOX2B mutations in retrotrapezoid cells decrease stimulation to the pacer cells located in the pre-Bötzinger complex region. • For idiopathic central hypoventilation, the etiology is unknown. • Opioid induces a dose-dependent respiratory rate depression by a combined inhibition (hyperpolarization) of pacer cells located in Pre-Bötzinger/Bötzinger complex and relay center parabrachial nucleus/Kolliker-Fuse complex.

Neuromuscular disorders ("cannot breathe")	• Motor neurons
	  ○ *Spinal cord injury (C3)*
	  ○ *Anterior horn cell (ALS, poliomyelitis)*
	• Peripheral neuropathy
	  ○ *Guillain–Barre*
	• Neuromuscular junction
	  ○ *Myasthenia gravis*
	  ○ *Eaton–Lambert*
	• Myopathies
		• The primary neuromuscular disorder affects the ability to translate ventilatory center output into appropriate action by the neuromuscular apparatus.

Chest wall abnormalities:	• Kyphoscoliosis • Morbid obesity • Pleural fibrosis • Thoracoplasty	• Increased work of breathing due to thoracic cage abnormalities, such as skeletal rigidity or excessive load from adipose tissue.
Lung disorders	• Chronic obstructive lung disease (COPD) • Advanced restrictive lung disease	• Mechanical effectiveness of ventilation is adversely affected by the underlying respiratory disease. Ultimately, the ventilatory control center undergoes adaptation, reducing the responsiveness to CO_2 in COPD. • In restrictive disorders, ventilatory drive remains high, but effectiveness is reduced by gas exchange abnormalities secondary to pulmonary parenchymal damage.

Abbreviations: ALS, amyotrophic lateral sclerosis, CO_2, carbon dioxide.

Initial Testing to Differentiate Chronic Hypercapnic Respiratory Failure Etiologies

Once the diagnosis of chronic hypercapnic respiratory failure is confirmed by arterial blood gas (ABG) or surrogate measures ($Paco_2 > 45$ mm Hg and elevated serum bicarbonate levels without any other cause for metabolic alkalosis), a clinical classification based on the patient's pulmonary function can be used to differentiate between various causes of respiratory failure.

Pulmonary function is often assessed by pulmonary function tests (PFTs). These tests can differentiate between anomalies in the ventilatory drive (respiratory control system) linked to normal PFTs, and abnormalities in pulmonary mechanics that result in abnormal PFTs[6] (**Fig. 1**, **Table 2**). Further narrowing of differential diagnoses may require additional testing, which will be covered in depth in the following sections (**Table 3**).

CLINICAL ASSESSMENT OF HYPERCAPNIC RESPIRATORY FAILURE BY DISORDERS
Obesity Hypoventilation Syndrome

According to the ICSD-3-TR, OHS is defined by obesity (BMI >30 kg/m^2) and daytime hypercapnia ($Paco_2 > 45$ mm Hg) that cannot be entirely attributed to an underlying cardiopulmonary or neurologic disorder (eg, lung parenchymal or airway disease, chest wall disorder, medication use, neuromuscular disorder).[4] OHS remains underdiagnosed in clinical practice in part due to a lack of specific signs and symptoms. Although the actual prevalence of the disease in the general adult population is unknown, estimates place it between 0.15% and 0.3%.[7] Prevalence is significantly higher in specific groups characterized by higher risk factors for OHS, such as obese individuals referred to sleep centers for evaluation of sleep-related breathing disorders (8%–20%) or morbidly obese patients referred for bariatric surgery (68.4%).[8,9] In the obstructive sleep apnea (OSA) population, there is a direct correlation between the severity of obesity and the prevalence of OHS. OHS is often associated with cardiopulmonary diseases (eg, pulmonary hypertension) and is linked to increased rates of mortality.[10]

History
Patients with OHS may present with one of two distinctive phenotypes: (1) OHS with OSA (OHS-OSA), which accounts for 90% of total OHS cases, with nearly 70% having severe OSA (apnea–hypopnea index ≥ 30 episodes per hour) and (2) 10% having sleep-dependent hypoventilation without OSA, also known as "true Pickwickian Syndrome."[11]

Compared to OSA without OHS, patients with OHS-OSA are older (50–60 years), with higher BMI (≥ 40 kg/m^2), and an equal prevalence in both genders.[12] These patients are also more likely to complain of daytime hypersomnolence and dyspnea, and they have a higher prevalence of hypertension and diabetes.[9] It should be noted that important racial differences may exist in this population. Asian individuals with OHS tend to be younger and they tend to develop OHS at lower BMIs than non-Asian populations.[13]

The group of individuals with OHS without OSA (true Pickwickian syndrome) is likely underdiagnosed and poorly characterized in the current literature. They are more likely to be older female individuals with characteristics similar to those with the OHS-OSA phenotype, with the distinction that witnessed apneas are less common.[14]

In stable conditions, undiagnosed patients with OHS may be referred to the sleep clinic with signs and symptoms indistinguishable from those of patients with eucapnic OSA (eg, loud snoring, witnessed apneas, nocturia, morning headaches, and excessive daytime sleepiness). When unstable, undiagnosed patients may initially seek medical attention due to acute-on-chronic (decompensated) hypercapnic respiratory failure, which is often mistakenly diagnosed as a COPD exacerbation. These patients typically require hospitalization, and their survival after discharge is correlated with initiating appropriate positive airway pressure therapy.[15,16]

Physical examination
Patients with OHS are often morbidly obese (BMI ≥ 40 kg/m^2). Physical examination findings may include plethora, an enlarged neck circumference, a crowded oropharynx, and scleral injection. Signs of pulmonary hypertension and/or right heart failure may be present, such as an elevated jugular venous pressure (>3 cm above the sternal angle), right ventricular heave by palpation, loud pulmonic valve closure (P2) on cardiac auscultation, and peripheral edema.[11]

Testing
When screening for OHS in obese patients suspected of having sleep-disordered breathing, pretest probability may guide the need to obtain ABG testing to measure ($Paco_2$). The pretest probability can be determined by the patient's BMI and the presence of signs and symptoms of OSA/OHS. Patients who have a high probability of having OHS (≥ 20%) share the following risk factors: severe obesity (BMI > 40 kg/m^2) along with typical signs and symptoms of OSA/OHS (eg, dyspnea, nocturia, lower extremity edema, excessive daytime

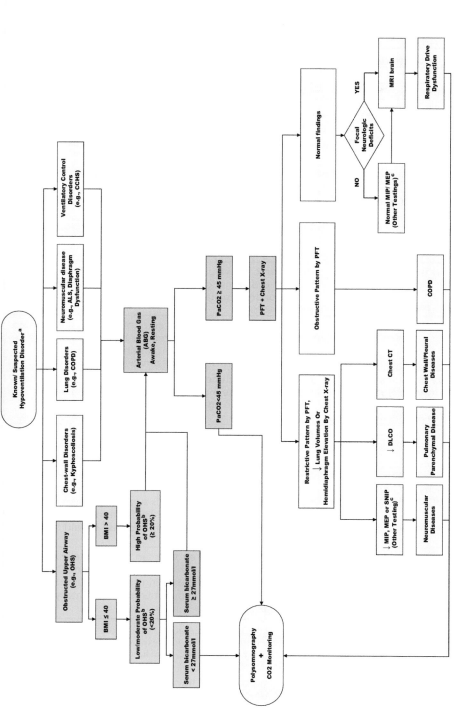

Fig. 1. Assessment of chronic hypercapnic respiratory failure. [a]See **Table 5** for signs and symptoms of chronic hypercapnic respiratory failure disorders. [b]High pretest probability of OHS: very symptomatic patients (e.g., dyspnea, sleepiness, lower extremity edema, daytime and/or nocturnal hypoxemia) with a BMI >40 kg/m2; Low or moderate pretest probability of OHS: less symptomatic patients with BMI 30–40 kg/m2. [c]See **Table 3**. Additional studies based on suspected etiology. *Abbreviations:* BMI, body mass index; CNS, central nervous system; COPD, chronic obstructive pulmonary disease; CXR, chest X-ray; CT chest, computed tomography; DLco, diffusing capacity for carbon monoxide; MEP, maximal expiratory pressure; MIP, maximal inspiratory pressure; MRI, magnetic resonance imaging; MVV, maximal voluntary ventilation; OHS, obesity hypoventilation syndrome; $PaCO_2$, partial pressure of carbon dioxide in arterial blood; PFT, pulmonary function tests; SNIP, sniff nasal inspiratory pressure.

Table 2
Pulmonary function test patterns and parameters in hypercapnic respiratory failure

	Obstructive Disease (eg, COPD)		Restrictive Disease (eg, NMD)
	FEV_1/FVC	FEV1 Percentage pred	VC or TLC Percentage pred
Pulmonary Function Test Patterns			
Normal	>70%	>80%	>80%
Mild	<70%	60%–80%	60%–80%
Moderate	<70%	40%–60%	50%–60%
Severe	<70%	<40%	<50%
↓ DLCO	Consider emphysema		Consider pulmonary parenchymal disease
↓ MIP/SNIP			Neuromuscular disease
		Interpretation	
Pulmonary Function Test Parameters			
Spirometry and lung volumes		Spirometry and lung volumes measurements can reveal patterns of volume and flow fluctuations, providing evidence of obstructive (eg, COPD) or restrictive (eg, NMD) physiology.	
Carbon monoxide diffusion capacity (DLCO)		DLCO can offer valuable information regarding changes in the gas exchange surface, such as emphysema, or the pulmonary vasculature, such as pulmonary hypertension.	
Vital capacity (VC)		VC represents the maximum amount of air that is exhaled after a full inspiration. It reflects inspiratory and expiratory muscle strength, respiratory system compliance (stiffness), and airways resistance.	
Maximal respiratory pressures (maximal inspiratory pressure [MIP], maximal expiratory pressure [MEP])		MIP and MEP can be used as markers of changes in the strength of the muscles involved in inhaling and exhaling when addressing neuromuscular diseases.	
sniff nasal inspiratory pressure (SNIP)		Measures inspiratory muscle strength and is complementary to MIP. Is useful in those patients where MIP cannot be performed due to oral weakness	
The difference between sitting and supine vital capacity (VC) or forced vital capacity (FVC)		The difference between sitting and supine VC or FVC can be used to support the diagnosis of diaphragmatic weakness or paralysis. This is suggested when VC (or FVC) decreases more than 20% from sitting to supine position. Physiologically, this decrease should be 5%–10%.	
Maximal voluntary ventilation (MVV)		MVV is the volume of air that can be maximally and rapidly inhaled and exhaled within 1 minute. It reflects both respiratory muscle strength and endurance, and it is typically reduced in patients with respiratory muscle weakness.	

Abbreviations: COPD, chronic obstructive pulmonary disease; DLCO, diffusion capacity; FEV1, forced expiratory volume in 1 second; FVC, forced vital capacity; MIP, maximal inspiratory pressure; MEP, maximal expiratory pressure; NMD, neuromuscular disease; pred, predicted value; SNIP, sniff nasal inspiratory pressure; TLC, total lung capacity.

sleepiness, fatigue, loud snoring, witnessed apneas) and mild hypoxemia during wakefulness and/or significant hypoxemia during sleep. These patients should proceed directly with ABG testing to confirm the suspected diagnosis of daytime hypercapnia. In contrast, for those patients with lower BMI (30–40 kg/m²) and low-to-moderate probability of having OHS (<20%), it is recommended to use serum bicarbonate level to decide whether to proceed to measure $Paco_2$ by ABG as the next step. In these patients, a serum bicarbonate level less than 27 mmol/L (64%–74% of obese patients with OSA) would likely permit forgoing ABG testing (high negative predictive value). On

Table 3
Additional studies based on suspected hypercapnic respiratory failure etiology

Testing	Ventilatory Control Disorders (eg, CCAHS)	Neuromuscular Disorders[a]	Lung/Chest Wall Disorders
$Paco_2$ (ABG or surrogate)	↑, or ↓ with voluntary hyperventilation	↑	↑
Chest radiograph or CT chest	N, or signs of pulmonary hypertension	N, low lung volumes, or hemidiaphragm elevation	N, or signs of underlying pulmonary disorder
Diaphragmatic fluoroscopy ("sniff test")	N	N, or paradoxic upward movement of hemidiaphragm	N
Diaphragmatic EMG	N	Abnormal	N
Nerve conduction studies	N	↓ or absence of phrenic nerve action potential	N
PFT and VC in both upright and supine positions	N	Restrictive, ΔVC more than 20% between upright and supine position	Restrictive (eg, kyphoscoliosis) or obstructive disorder (eg, COPD)
MIP/MEP	N	↓	N
Maximal sniff nasal inspiratory pressure (SNIP)	N	↓	N
Polysomnography	• Hypoventilation with sustained oxyhemoglobin desaturations, worsen during slow wave sleep, less in REM. • Central apneas may be present.	• Hypoventilation with sustained oxyhemoglobin desaturations, worse in REM. • Central or obstructive apneas may be present.	• Hypoventilation with sustained oxyhemoglobin desaturations, worse in REM

Abbreviations: COPD, chronic obstructive pulmonary disease; CT chest, computed tomography of chest; EMG, electromyography; MEP, maximal expiratory pressure; MIP, maximal inspiratory pressure; N, normal; $Paco_2$, partial pressure of carbon dioxide in arterial blood; PFT, pulmonary function test; REM, rapid eye movement; SNIP; maximal sniff nasal inspiratory pressure; VC, vital capacity.
[a] Respiratory motor neurons, spinal cord, phrenic nerves, respiratory muscles.

the contrary, ABG analysis is recommended in those with serum bicarbonate ≥ 27 mmol/L (26%–36% of obese patients with OSA[17]; **Fig. 1**).

According to the alveolar gas equation, hypoxemia can result from hypercapnia. An overnight pulse oximetry test showing a sustained low baseline O_2 saturation could be used as a surrogate indicator of hypercapnia. However, because hypoxemia may manifest in morbidly obese patients in the absence of hypercapnia due to other factors (eg, atelectasis), overnight oximetry is not currently recommended as a single screening tool to guide the need for ABG testing in a patient with suspected OHS.[17]

Based on the ICSD-3-TR definition, polysomnography (PSG) is not required for the diagnosis of OHS. However, laboratory-based PSG is commonly performed to identify the nature of the sleep-related breathing disorder present and to individualize positive airway pressure therapy.

Results of additional tests in patients with OHS may be indistinguishable from other causes of chronic hypercapnia with subsequent hypoxemia (eg, secondary polycythemia, elevated pulmonary arterial pressures, and right heart failure on echocardiogram). Because OHS is a diagnosis of exclusion, individualized testing to rule out other causes of chronic hypercapnia in adults is required (eg, COPD, neuromuscular weakness, hypothyroidism, advanced interstitial lung disease, and chronic narcotic use).[4]

Chronic Obstructive Pulmonary Disease and Overlap Syndrome

COPD is commonly associated with a broad spectrum of sleep-related breathing disorders such as sleep-related hypoxemia, sleep-related hypoventilation, and OSA.

The prevalence of sleep-related hypoventilation varies in relation to the severity of COPD. In those patients with mild COPD and normal awake ABGs, the prevalence of nocturnal hypoventilation may be low (6%–10%) and limited to REM sleep. In contrast, the prevalence may be high (43%) and sustained throughout sleep in those with more severe COPD and awake hypercapnia.[18]

COPD and OSA are highly prevalent chronic diseases that frequently coexist, a condition known as overlap syndrome. Because the mortality associated with overlap syndrome is higher than the mortality associated with either COPD or OSA alone, it is important to screen for OSA early in patients with COPD.[19]

History

Some COPD-related features may predispose to or protect against OSA. In patients with COPD with predominantly emphysematous changes, features such as underweight, hyperinflation associated with a low diaphragmatic position, and decreased REM sleep may decrease the likelihood of OSA. On the other hand, in patients with COPD with a predominately chronic bronchitis phenotype, the presence of weight gain, cigarette smoking, rostral fluid shifts while supine, medications (eg, chronic corticosteroid use), and higher diaphragmatic position can predispose to OSA.[20]

In comparison to COPD without OSA, patients with overlap syndrome are male predominant, have a higher BMI, a more extensive history of smoking, a higher number of cardiovascular comorbidities (eg, ischemic cardiomyopathy, hypertension), and experience more frequent COPD exacerbations requiring hospitalization.[21]

In contrast to patients with OSA without COPD, those with overlap syndrome typically experience less prominent OSA symptoms (eg, snoring, witnessed apneas, unrefreshing sleep, and daytime sleepiness) and have a higher prevalence and severity of hypoxemia and pulmonary hypertension.[22] In addition to sleep complaints, patients with undiagnosed COPD will also report daytime respiratory symptoms such as dyspnea and a persistent productive cough.

Physical examination

In patients with established COPD, the presence of obesity (BMI $\geq$ 30 kg/m^2) and cardiovascular disease places them at high risk for overlap syndrome. Physical examination may reveal a large neck circumference, audible wheezing, an enlarged (barrel) chest, cyanosis, and findings of pulmonary hypertension or cor pulmonale, such as peripheral edema.

Testing

According to the latest guidelines from the American Thoracic Society, individuals with chronic stable hypercapnic COPD (with a spirometric ratio of <0.70 and resting $Paco_2$ levels above 45 mm Hg, but not during an exacerbation) should be screened for OSA before starting long-term noninvasive ventilation (NIV) therapy.[23] Commonly used screening questionnaires for OSA, such as the STOP-BANG questionnaire can be used as the first step in those patients with COPD with suspected OSA symptoms. Patients with a positive screen result should undergo laboratory-based PSG to assess OSA and customize positive airway pressure titration.[23]

Overnight oximetry is occasionally ordered in patients with COPD to screen for sleep-related breathing disorders. The pattern of O_2 desaturation may differ between patients with COPD, OSA, and overlap syndrome. In COPD without OSA, periods of sustained nocturnal desaturation are observed, being more pronounced during REM sleep. The severity of nocturnal desaturation typically correlates with the baseline oxygen saturation level while awake. In OSA without COPD, intermittent (brief) desaturations usually revert to a normal baseline saturation level between apneic events. In patients with COPD–OSA overlap, episodic desaturation also develops, typically from a low saturation baseline, and worsens during periods of REM sleep. Although overnight pulse oximetry in overlap syndrome may show a lower baseline O_2 saturation and more pronounced desaturation compared to OSA without COPD, it is not recommended as a screening test as it is not sensitive, and it does not provide information on the degree of hypoventilation.

In-laboratory PSG is the gold standard method used to diagnose sleep apnea events (obstructive and central sleep apnea), and/or sleep-related hypoventilation in patients with COPD. During the study, CO_2 levels can be measured using invasive and noninvasive techniques, by monitoring $ETCO_2$ or $TcCO_2$ tension.

In patients with established OSA and suspected COPD (eg, dyspnea on exertion, wheezing, chronic cough, and sputum production), the diagnosis of obstructive lung disease requires a spirometry test. This test measures the airflow limitation in the lungs by assessing the ratio of forced expiratory volume in one second to forced vital capacity (FEV1/FVC). A ratio below 0.7 or below the lower limit of normal indicates the presence of airflow limitation (see **Table 2**). Frequently, an additional test, such as an ABG or venous blood gas, is obtained to evaluate the extent of hypercapnia.

Respiratory Muscle Weakness from Neuromuscular Diseases

NMDs are neurologic disorders that compromise muscle function directly or indirectly by affecting nerves or neuromuscular junctions. Respiratory muscle weakness (RMW) is a potentially life-threatening condition defined as the persistent incapacity of respiratory muscles to perform their mechanical "pump" functions. Nocturnal hypoventilation may be the initial manifestation of various NMDs, some of which may have limited signs of non-RMW. Early detection of respiratory failure is critical, as it may serve as a diagnostic and prognostic indicator, and its early treatment may improve survival[24] (**Table 4**).

History

Awake symptoms of dyspnea are often present late in the disease and are limited to the patient's activity level. Diaphragmatic weakness may present with orthopnea when lying down, and intercostal muscle weakness may cause dyspnea when upright. Those patients with bulbar dysfunction may complain of speech and swallowing difficulties, weak cough, or the sensation of choking when lying down.

Table 4
Neuromuscular disorders associated with respiratory muscle weakness

Mechanism	Diseases
Spinal lesion	• Demyelinating disease (eg, multiple sclerosis) • Spinal infarct/hemorrhage • Spinal inflammation (eg, transverse myelitis)
Motor nerve dysfunction	• Amyotrophic lateral sclerosis (ALS) • Cervical spondylosis • Guillain–Barre syndrome • Poliomyelitis • Phrenic nerve injury • Neural sarcoidosis
Neuromuscular junction dysfunction	• Myasthenia gravis • Lambert–Eaton syndrome
Myopathy	• Muscular dystrophy • Myotonic dystrophy • Mitochondrial myopathy • Malnutrition • Polymyositis/ dermatomyositis

Patient with NMD may complain of restless and unrefreshing sleep, vivid dreams, daytime somnolence, lethargy, poor concentration, and impaired cognition or affect. Some of these symptoms may be indistinguishable from OSA. Hypercapnia-related symptoms usually present later in the progression of respiratory failure. Those symptoms may include headache that is worse on waking, poor appetite, confusion, and daytime drowsiness.

Physical examination

Besides signs and symptoms from the underlying NMD (eg, muscle atrophy, fasciculation, hyper/hyporeflexia), clinical signs of RMW include rapid shallow breathing, use of accessory muscles, reduced chest expansion, reduced breath sounds, abdominal paradox (inward movement of the abdomen on inspiration), and weak cough and sniff. Signs of intercostal muscle weakness with preserved diaphragmatic function (eg, spinal muscular atrophy) include bell-shaped chest deformity and paradoxic breathing (inward chest wall movement on inspiration and outward on expiration). Scoliosis, with evidence of surgical correction, might be present, particularly in childhood-onset NMD. Signs of respiratory failure include central cyanosis, tremors, dilated veins, bounding pulse, papilledema, confusion, and drowsiness (**Table 5**).

Testing

Respiratory symptoms caused by RMW may only become evident during the later stages of the disease when there has been a significant decline in respiratory muscle strength. Early diagnosis and intervention can enhance the chances of survival for certain neuromuscular disorders. However, the frequency of assessments and testing may vary depending on the disease's progression rate.

It is recommended to perform periodic testing, such as ABG analysis, PFTs, and muscle strength assessments, in the diagnosis and in assessing the prognosis of RMW.[24] If there is a suspicion of diaphragmatic dysfunction, it may be appropriate to begin with nonspecific radiologic investigations, such as the fluoroscopic sniff test. If radiologic results are inconclusive, it is advisable to undertake specialized diaphragmatic testing (see **Table 3**).

- Awake ABG values should be obtained to assess the degree of hypoventilation and hypoxemia. During the early stages of the disease process, it is possible to observe normal levels of $Paco_2$ during wakefulness, with hypercapnia confined to sleep periods. Chronic compensated respiratory acidosis

Table 5
Signs and symptoms of chronic hypercapnic respiratory failure by disorders

	History and Symptoms	Physical Examination Findings
Chest wall abnormalities (eg, kyphoscoliosis)	• History of spinal or pleural disorders • Dyspnea on exertion • Decreased physical exercise endurance	• Thoracic cage deformities (eg, pectus excavatum), spinal deformities (eg, scoliosis, kyphosis, surgical scars)
Obstructive lung diseases (eg, COPD)	• Dyspnea • Chronic cough • Sputum production • History of smoking	• Barrel chest • Wheezing • Clubbing and cyanosis
Neuromuscular disorders (eg, ALS)	• Weak cough • Dyspnea • Orthopnea • Bulbar dysfunction[a] • Choking during sleep • Focal neurologic deficits • History of spinal cord injuries	• Cranial nerve dysfunctions • Upper motor neural lesions[b] • Lower motor neural lesions[c] • Thoracoabdominal paradox (eg, diaphragm dysfunction) • Rapid shallow breathing • Accessory respiratory muscle use
Ventilatory control abnormalities (eg, CCHS)	• Witnessed apneas • Excessive daytime sleepiness • Paroxysmal nocturnal dyspnea • Signs of cranial nerve deficits in brainstem disorders • History of medications or substance use or abuse	• Disease-specific findings

Abbreviations: ALS, amyotrophic lateral sclerosis; CCHS, congenital central alveolar hypoventilation syndrome; COPD, chronic obstructive pulmonary disease.
  [a] Drooling, dysarthria, dysphagia, facial or tongue weakness, nasal speech.
  [b] Increased muscle tone (spasticity, spastic paralysis), increased deep tendon reflexes (hyper-reflexia), upgoing plantar reflex (Babinski sign).
  [c] Reduced muscle tone (muscle atrophy) and strength (flaccid paralysis), denervation (fasciculations), decreased deep tendon reflexes (hyporeflexia), downgoing plantar reflex.

may develop over time if there is a progression of RMW.

• Spirometry and lung volumes measurements will characterize the severity of the restrictive pulmonary pattern (see **Table 2**). Given the repeatability of spirometry results over time, its most significant value is in the longitudinal assessment of the NMD progression. Patients with neuromuscular junction disorder such as myasthenia gravis or Lambert–Eaton syndrome may have fluctuation of muscle weakness. Therefore, several tests with a stable trend rather than a single study might be required for these disorders. Patients with suspected diaphragmatic dysfunction should undergo a measure of vital capacity (VC) or FVC in both upright and supine positions. A discrepancy of VC (or FVC) of more than 20% across postures is highly suggestive of diaphragmatic weakness and nocturnal hypoventilation.[25]

• Respiratory muscle strength is commonly measured by static mouth pressures, such as maximal inspiratory (MIP) and expiratory pressures (MEP), or dynamic pressures, such as sniff nasal inspiratory pressure (SNIP). MIP and MEP reflect the strength of inspiratory (predominately diaphragm) and expiratory muscles, respectively.[26] A MIP below one-third of normal predicts hypercapnic respiratory failure (normal values are more negative than −60 cm H_2O). SNIP measures inspiratory muscle function, mainly diaphragmatic muscle strength, and it is particularly useful when MIP cannot be obtained due to significant weakness (eg, bulbar dysfunction with weak lip seal around mouthpieces or submaximal efforts). An SNIP greater than 70 cm H_2O (in men) or greater than 60 cm H_2O (in women) usually excludes significant RMW. SNIP may also predict nocturnal hypoventilation and respiratory failure in

ALS, and an SNIP that is 35% of normal value ($\sim$ <40 cm H_2O) requires the initiation of NIV.

- Diaphragmatic testing: While static radiologic testing (eg, chest radiograph or computed tomography scan of the chest) may show elevation of one or both hemidiaphragms and small lung volumes, dynamic fluoroscopic testing during a sniff maneuver (sniff testing) may detect no movement (or paradoxic movement) of a hemidiaphragm, supporting the diagnosis of diaphragmatic paralysis. When radiologic results are equivocal, specific diaphragmatic testing should be considered, such as phrenic nerve conduction studies combined with diaphragmatic electromyography or diaphragmatic ultrasonography to assess the muscle contractile response to stimulation.

- Nocturnal testing may include an overnight oximetry and/or a laboratory-based PSG. Nocturnal oximetry is a cost-effective and widely available method to detect episodes of sustained nocturnal desaturation, which may precede a decrease in VC.[27] Although laboratory-based PSG is not required to initiate NIV therapy in these patients, it is still considered the gold standard for assessing sleep-disordered breathing, including sleep-related hypoventilation, and it can assist in the optimization of nocturnal NIV.

Congenital Central Hypoventilation Syndrome

Congenital central hypoventilation syndrome (CCHS), commonly known as "Ondine's curse," is a rare autosomal dominant genetic disorder characterized by sleep-related hypoventilation, usually at birth, otherwise unexplained by a primary pulmonary, neurologic, or metabolic disease. It is caused by monoallelic mutations of pairedlike homeobox 2B gene (PHOX2B) on chromosome 4p12.[28] The reported incidence of CCHS is one in every 148,000 to 200,000 live births, and it is classified into 2 types based on the time of onset and severity of symptoms.

1. Neonatal-onset CCHS (within the first 30 days of life) is characterized by hypoventilation with monotonous respiratory rate.
2. Late-onset CCHS is less common than neonatal-onset CCHS. It may present phenotypically later in life, even in adulthood, with less severe symptoms.

The neuroanatomical pathway resulting in central hypoventilation in humans is not well characterized. In animal models, neurons in the retrotrapezoid nucleus located in the medulla function as central chemoreceptors (CO_2/H^+) and provide excitatory neurotransmission via glutamate to the pre-Bötzinger complex region, which serves as a central controller of respiration. PHOX2B mutations in cells of the retrotrapezoid nucleus in mice result in central hypoventilation, apnea, and a reduced or absent ventilatory responsiveness to CO_2.[29]

History

Although patients with CCHS typically present as sporadic cases (due to de novo mutations), family clusters may be identified (autosomal dominant inheritance pattern). It is equally distributed among genders and ethnic/racial groups.

In addition to alveolar hypoventilation, patients with CCHS may have a history of Hirschsprung's disease (delayed passage of meconium, constipation, abdominal distension, tight anal sphincter, or symptoms of enterocolitis), autonomic nervous system dysfunction (abnormal thermoregulation, altered gastrointestinal dysmotility, and altered pain perception), cardiac arrhythmias (decreased heart rate variability), and neural crest tumors (neuroblastomas).

In neonatal-onset CCHS, affected infants present with cyanosis, shallow breathing, and central apneas occurring during sleep. Owing to their lack of ventilatory response to hypercapnia or hypoxemia, patients do not typically show signs of increased respiratory distress (such as nasal flaring, tachypnea, or chest retractions). As a result, diagnosis may be delayed, and the patient's initial presentation may be a cardiopulmonary arrest. After confirmation of alveolar hypoventilation, most neonates with CCHS require intubation and mechanical ventilation, with subsequent difficulties usually encountered in trying to wean invasive ventilatory support.

In late-onset CCHS, patients may present with episodes of cyanosis, cor pulmonale, unexplained seizures, or unusual degrees of respiratory depression after anesthesia (unable to be extubated), minor respiratory infections, or in response to sedatives or anticonvulsant drugs. These patients may also present later in life with unexplained pulmonary hypertension.

Testing

The infant with hypoventilation should undergo a thorough evaluation for primary respiratory, cardiac, or neurologic disorders that can cause hypoventilation (see **Tables 1** and **5**). This is achieved through multidisciplinary collaboration involving pediatric pulmonologists, neurologists, and geneticists. Chest radiography, airway endoscopy, electrocardiogram and echocardiogram, MRI of the brain, diaphragm ultrasound or fluoroscopy, metabolic studies, and comprehensive neurologic evaluation are often required.[30]

- ABG will support the diagnosis of nocturnal alveolar hypoventilation based on elevated $Paco_2$ during sleep. $Paco_2$ during wakefulness may be normal or elevated, depending on the severity of respiratory failure.
- A molecular genetic testing panel should be undertaken if a basic evaluation/testing of more common causes of hypoventilation does not suggest an alternative diagnosis. As an initial test, the PHOX2B screening test may detect up to 95% of PHOX2B gene mutations. There are 2 types of PHOX2B genotype variants: polyalanine repeat expansion mutations (PARMs) and nonpolyalanine repeat expansion mutations (NPARMs). Approximately 90% of reported cases are polyalanine repeat expansion mutations (PARMs) in exon 3. The severity of ventilatory defect is higher in those patients with NPARM and those with longer PARM and NPARM sequences. If the PHOX2B screening test is negative, but there is still a high clinical suspicion, sequencing the coding region of the PHOX2B gene will detect 99% of mutations.
- In children with suspected nocturnal hypoventilation, PSG with CO_2 monitoring should be conducted. In pediatric patients, hypoventilation is defined as an elevation of $Paco_2$ (or surrogate) greater than 50 mm Hg for more than 25% of total sleep duration.[4,5] In patients with CCHS, hypoventilation and hypoxemia are more severe in NREM sleep than in REM sleep, in contrast to most other forms of sleep-disordered breathing. In the PSG, a decrease in breathing depth and rate and a decrease in arousal response to hypoxemia and hypercapnia can be observed.[5]

SUMMARY

Chronic hypercapnic respiratory failure, defined as an elevation in the arterial carbon dioxide tension, may be encountered during the evaluation of sleep-related breathing disorders. Underdiagnosed, the signs and symptoms of chronic hypercapnic respiratory failure may be nonspecific, with sleep disruption and daytime impairment being prevalent. A comprehensive clinical history, a thorough physical examination, and a systematic testing approach are critical to establish the etiology.

DISCLOSURE

The authors have no conflict of interest to declare.

REFERENCES

1. Roussos C, Koutsoukou A. Respiratory failure. Review. Eur Respir J 2003;47(Supplement):3s–14s.
2. Douglas NJ, White DP, Pickett CK, et al. Respiration during sleep in normal man. Thorax 1982;37(11): 840–4.
3. Midgren B, Hansson L. Changes in transcutaneous PCO2 with sleep in normal subjects and in patients with chronic respiratory diseases. Eur J Respir Dis 1987;71(5):388–94.
4. International classification of sleep disorders. 3rd edition Text Revision. Darien, IL 2023: American Academy of Sleep Medicine; 2023.
5. Berry RB, Quan SF, Abreu AR, et al. The AASM manual for the scoring of sleep and associated events: rules, terminology and technical specifications. Version 2.6. 2020. Available at: https://aasm.org/resources/pdf/scoring-manual-preface.pdf.
6. Pellegrino R, Viegi G, Brusasco V, et al. Interpretative strategies for lung function tests. Eur Respir J 2005;26(5):948–68.
7. Mokhlesi B. Obesity hypoventilation syndrome: a state-of-the-art review. Respir Care 2010;55(10): 1347–62 [discussion 1363-5].
8. Kaw R, Hernandez AV, Walker E, et al. Determinants of hypercapnia in obese patients with obstructive sleep apnea: a systematic review and metaanalysis of cohort studies. Chest 2009;136(3):787–96.
9. Tran K, Wang L, Gharaibeh S, et al. Elucidating predictors of obesity hypoventilation syndrome in a large bariatric surgery cohort. Ann Am Thorac Soc 2020;17(10):1279–88.
10. Castro-Añón O, Pérez de Llano LA, De la Fuente Sánchez S, et al. Obesity-hypoventilation syndrome: increased risk of death over sleep apnea syndrome. PLoS One 2015;10(2):e0117808.
11. Masa JF, Corral J, Alonso ML, et al. Efficacy of different treatment alternatives for obesity hypoventilation syndrome. Pickwick study. Am J Respir Crit Care Med 2015;192(1):86–95.
12. Palm A, Midgren B, Janson C, et al. Gender differences in patients starting long-term home mechanical ventilation due to obesity hypoventilation syndrome. Respir Med 2016;110:73–8.
13. Akashiba T, Akahoshi T, Kawahara S, et al. Clinical characteristics of obesity-hypoventilation syndrome in Japan: a multi-center study. Intern Med 2006; 45(20):1121–5.
14. Masa JF, Corral J, Caballero C, et al. Non-invasive ventilation in obesity hypoventilation syndrome without severe obstructive sleep apnoea. Thorax 2016;71(10):899–906.
15. Marik PE, Chen C. The clinical characteristics and hospital and post-hospital survival of patients with the obesity hypoventilation syndrome: analysis of a large cohort. Obesity science & practice 2016;2(1):40–7.

16. Mokhlesi B, Masa JF, Afshar M, et al. The effect of hospital discharge with empiric noninvasive ventilation on mortality in hospitalized patients with obesity hypoventilation syndrome. An individual patient data meta-analysis. Ann Am Thorac Soc 2020;17(5): 627–37.

17. Mokhlesi B, Masa JF, Brozek JL, et al. Evaluation and management of obesity hypoventilation syndrome. An official American Thoracic Society Clinical Practice Guideline. Am J Respir Crit Care Med 2019;200(3):e6–24.

18. O'Donoghue FJ, Catcheside PG, Ellis EE, et al. Sleep hypoventilation in hypercapnic chronic obstructive pulmonary disease: prevalence and associated factors. Eur Respir J 2003;21(6):977–84.

19. Starr P, Agarwal A, Singh G, et al. Obstructive sleep apnea with chronic obstructive pulmonary disease among medicare beneficiaries. Ann Am Thorac Soc 2019;16(1):153–6.

20. Biselli P, Grossman PR, Kirkness JP, et al. The effect of increased lung volume in chronic obstructive pulmonary disease on upper airway obstruction during sleep. J Appl Physiol (1985) 2015;119(3):266–71.

21. Steveling EH, Clarenbach CF, Miedinger D, et al. Predictors of the overlap syndrome and its association with comorbidities in patients with chronic obstructive pulmonary disease. Respiration 2014; 88(6):451–7.

22. Kendzerska T, Leung RS, Aaron SD, et al. Cardiovascular outcomes and all-cause mortality in patients with obstructive sleep apnea and chronic obstructive pulmonary disease (overlap syndrome). Ann Am Thorac Soc 2019;16(1):71–81.

23. Macrea M, Oczkowski S, Rochwerg B, et al. Long-term noninvasive ventilation in chronic stable hypercapnic chronic obstructive pulmonary disease. An official American Thoracic Society Clinical Practice Guideline. Am J Respir Crit Care Med 2020;202(4): e74–87.

24. Khan A, Frazer-Green L, Amin R, et al. Respiratory management of patients with neuromuscular weakness: an American College of Chest Physicians Clinical Practice guideline and Expert panel report. Chest 2023;164(2):394–413.

25. Allen SM, Hunt B, Green M. Fall in vital capacity with posture. Br J Dis Chest 1985;79(3):267–71.

26. ATS/ERS Statement on respiratory muscle testing. Am J Respir Crit Care Med 2002;166(4):518–624.

27. Kelly CR, Parra-Cantu C, Thapa P, et al. Comparative performance of different respiratory test parameters for detection of early respiratory insufficiency in patients with ALS. Neurology 2022;99(7):e743–50.

28. Weese-Mayer DE, Rand CM, Zhou A, et al. Congenital central hypoventilation syndrome: a bedside-to-bench success story for advancing early diagnosis and treatment and improved survival and quality of life. Pediatr Res 2017;81(1–2):192–201.

29. Nattie E. Ondine undone. N Engl J Med 2015;373(6): 573–5.

30. Weese-Mayer DE, Berry-Kravis EM, Ceccherini I, et al. An official ATS clinical policy statement: congenital central hypoventilation syndrome: genetic basis, diagnosis, and management. Am J Respir Crit Care Med 2010;181(6):626–44.

Chronic Obstructive Pulmonary Disease and Obstructive Sleep Apnea Overlap Syndrome
An Update on the Epidemiology, Pathophysiology, and Management

Benjamin H.M. Nguyen, MBBS, FRACP[a,b,c,d,*],
Patrick B. Murphy, MBBS, PhD, MRCP[e,f], Brendon J. Yee, MBChB, FRACP, PhD[b,d]

KEYWORDS

- Comorbidity • Epidemiology • Exacerbations • Mortality • Management
- Positive airway pressure therapy

KEY POINTS

- Overlap syndrome (OVS) is common and should be considered as a potential diagnosis when reviewing patients with either chronic obstructive pulmonary disease (COPD) or obstructive sleep apnea (OSA), as the combination is frequently missed.
- Classical risk factors for OSA may not be reliable in patients with COPD and clinicians should consider sleep studies in patients with COPD who are overweight, have comorbid cardiovascular disease and/or frequent exacerbations despite maximal therapy.
- Patients with OVS have an increased risk of hospitalization and mortality compared to patients with COPD alone.
- In patients with OVS, treatment with continuous positive airway pressure may improve symptoms and reduce hospitalization rates and excess mortality.

INTRODUCTION

The co-occurrence of COPD and OSA termed the "overlap syndrome" (OVS) was first coined by Flenley in 1985.[1] Despite being recognized almost 40 years ago, it remains an under-researched area.[2,3] Part of the reason is that studies involving patients with chronic obstructive pulmonary disease (COPD) often exclude patients with obstructive sleep apnea (OSA) and similarly, OSA studies typically exclude patients with concomitant respiratory disease. COPD is a chronic inflammatory condition characterized by airflow limitation, gas

[a] Department of Thoracic Medicine, Level 4 Xavier Building, St Vincent's Hospital, 390 Victoria Street, Darlinghurst, NSW 2010, Australia; [b] Department of Respiratory and Sleep Medicine, Royal Prince Alfred Hospital, Level 11 Royal Prince Alfred Hospital, Missenden Road, Camperdown, NSW 2050, Australia; [c] Faculty of Medicine and Health, Sydney Medical School, Sydney Medical School Central Sydney, The University of Sydney, NSW 2006, Australia; [d] The Woolcock Institute of Medical Research, Macquarie University, 2 Innovation Road, Macquarie Park, NSW 2113, Australia; [e] Lane Fox Respiratory Service, Division of Heart, Lung and Critical Care, Guy's & St Thomas NHS Foundation Trust, Ground Floor, South Wing, St Thomas' Hospital, Westminster Bridge Road, London SE1 7EH; [f] King's College London, Strand, London WC2R 2LS, United Kingdon
* Corresponding author. Department of Thoracic Medicine, Level 4, St Vincents Hospital, 390 Victoria Street, Darlinghurst, NSW 2010, Australia.
E-mail address: Benjamin.nguyen@svha.org.au

Sleep Med Clin 19 (2024) 405–417
https://doi.org/10.1016/j.jsmc.2024.04.003
1556-407X/24/© 2024 Elsevier Inc. All rights reserved.

trapping, and lung hyperinflation, which is usually associated with exposure to noxious particles or gases, typically cigarette smoke.[4] OSA is the most common sleep-related breathing disorder, occurring as a result of repetitive upper airway collapse during sleep resulting in hypoxia, hypercapnia, and sleep fragmentation.[5] Observational studies suggest that when both conditions coexist, it is associated with greater morbidity and mortality compared to either COPD or OSA alone.[6–10] This review examines the complex interactions between COPD and OSA and summarizes the latest evidence for treatment of OVS.

PREVALENCE OF OVERLAP SYNDROME

The prevalence of OVS in the general population has been estimated to be between 1% and 3.6%.[8] However, prevalence estimates of OVS in COPD or OSA cohorts are significantly higher and vary substantially between studies. In studies that used spirometry and polysomnography (PSG), the prevalence of OVS varies widely, between 10% and 78% in COPD cohorts and 11% to 56% in OSA cohorts (**Table 1**).[8,11,12] These discrepant findings are likely due in part to selection bias, with studies using different cohorts in different countries. Additionally, many of the studies were not designed with the primary aim of assessing the prevalence of OVS. For instance, 2 studies that reported an OVS prevalence of greater than 50% included only patients hospitalized with COPD who may be more likely to desaturate during sleep, thus overestimating the apnea–hypopnea index (AHI).[13,14] There were also inconsistent definitions of OSA between studies, with AHI thresholds ranging between 5 and 15/h, highlighting the lack of consensus on a definition of OVS.[8–10]

RELATIONSHIP BETWEEN OBSTRUCTIVE SLEEP APNEA AND CHRONIC OBSTRUCTIVE PULMONARY DISEASE

There are conflicting reports regarding the relationship between COPD severity and the presence of OSA. Sanders and colleagues analyzed 1132 patients with COPD from the Sleep Heart Health Study, a multicenter cohort study aimed at assessing the relationship between sleep disordered breathing and cardiovascular disease (CVD) in adults.[15] They also assessed the prevalence of OSA in patients with a forced expiratory volume in 1 s (FEV1)/forced vital capacity (FVC) ratio of less than 0.7 and those with an FEV1/FVC ratio of greater than 0.7 and found that there was no difference between groups. The participants in this

study represented a community population and had overall mild airflow obstruction. However, in patients with moderate-to-severe COPD, the prevalence of OSA has been demonstrated to be as high as 66%, suggesting that OVS may be more common with increasing COPD severity.[16] The participants in this observational study were recruited from a pulmonary rehabilitation program and had a mean FEV1 of 43% predicted, while over one-third were prescribed domiciliary oxygen. In contrast to these findings, Steveling and colleagues analyzed 177 patients with stable COPD and found no correlation between Global Initiative for Chronic Obstructive Lung Disease stages and AHI.[17] Body mass index (BMI) was found to be an independent predictor of AHI severity and patients with severe COPD in this study tended to have a lower AHI. Indeed, patients with advanced emphysema and lung hyperinflation are typically underweight and are thought to have less collapsible upper airways due to increased lung volumes and increased caudal traction on the trachea.[18–20] The presence of emphysema and gas trapping in smokers with OSA has also been shown to be inversely correlated with the AHI.[21]

PATHOPHYSIOLOGY

A number of physiologic changes that normally occur during sleep can compromise the respiratory system in patients with COPD, including reduced respiratory drive, reduced respiratory muscle activity (particularly during rapid eye movement [REM] sleep), and impaired lung mechanics.[22–24] Douglas and colleagues demonstrated a reduction in minute ventilation in normal subjects during all stages of sleep compared to wakefulness.[22] These changes were most pronounced during REM sleep, where tidal volumes dropped by 73% compared to wakefulness. The reduction in tidal volume was only partially offset by a corresponding increase in respiratory frequency. This partial compensatory response can be explained by the diminished ventilatory responses to both hypoxia and hypercapnia observed during sleep.[25–27] Furthermore, changes in lung mechanics occur in the supine posture due to upward displacement of the diaphragm, resulting in reduced functional residual capacity, and worsening ventilation perfusion mismatch, and nocturnal hypoxia.[24,28] While these changes may have minimal impact on healthy individuals, they are accentuated in patients with COPD.[29] Jolley and colleagues measured diaphragm electromyography during wakefulness in patients with COPD and found these individuals needed to

Table 1
Prevalence studies of overlap syndrome

Author Year	Country	Study Population	Method of Recruitment	Mean Age (years), Male %	AHI	Prevalence of OVS
Bednarek et al,[92] 2005	Poland	General population (n = 676)	Random sample	52% male	AHI >5	1%
Sanders et al,[15] 2003	USA	General population (n = 5954)	Random sample from Sleep Heart Health study	Age 63, 47% male	AHI >15	2.7%
Chaouat et al,[93] 1995	France	OSA patients (n = 265)	Consecutive sleep lab patients	Age 54, 92% male	AHI >20	11%
Shiina et al,[94] 2012	Japan	OSA patients (n = 524)	Consecutive sleep lab patients	Age 50, 100% male	AHI ≥5	12%
Rizzi et al,[95] 1997	Italy	OSA patients (n = 168)	Consecutive sleep lab patients	Age 56, 85% male	AHI >15	19.5%
López-Acevedo et al,[96] 2009	Puerto Rico	OSA patients (n = 52)	Consecutive sleep lab patients		AHI >5 with symptoms or AHI >15 without symptoms	55.7%
Perimenis et al,[97] 2007	Greece	COPD patients (n = 720)	Consecutive outpatients with COPD	100% male	AHI >5 with symptoms	10.3%
Machado et al,[6] 2010	Brazil	COPD patients (n = 603)	Consecutive COPD patients requiring LTOT		AHI >15	15.7%
Zhou et al,[54] 2020	China	COPD patients (n = 151)	Consecutive outpatients with COPD		AHI ≥5	16.60%
Steveling et al,[17] 2014	Switzerland	COPD patients (n = 177)	Consecutive outpatients with COPD	Age 64, 63% male	AHI >10	19%
Zhang et al,[98] 2022	China	COPD patients (n = 842)	Random sample of outpatients with COPD	Age 63, 72% male	AHI ≥5	23.0%
Zeng et al,[99] 2022	China	COPD patients (n = 886)	Consecutive outpatients with COPD	Age 67, 90% male	AHI ≥15	29.8%
Wang et al,[100] 2020	China	COPD patients (n = 277)	Consecutive outpatients with COPD	Age 67, 85% male	AHI ≥15	38.30%

(continued on next page)

Table 1
(continued)

Author Year	Country	Study Population	Method of Recruitment	Mean Age (years), Male %	AHI	Prevalence of OVS
Zhang et al,[101] 2019	China	COPD patients (n = 73)	Consecutive outpatients with COPD	Age 66, 78% male	AHI ≥15	43.80%
Zhang et al,[102] 2020	China	COPD patients (n = 65)	Consecutive outpatients with COPD	Age 70, 83% male	AHI ≥15	44.60%
Climaco et al,[103] 2022	Brazil	COPD patients (n = 102)	Consecutive outpatients with COPD	Age 69, 69% male	AHI ≥15	50.0%
Wu et al,[104] 2020	China	COPD patients (n = 116)	Consecutive outpatients with COPD	Age 62, 93% male	AHI ≥5	53.40%
Yang et al,[105] 2020	China	COPD patients (n = 124)	Consecutive outpatients with COPD	Age 70, 57% male	AHI ≥5	56.40%
Soler et al,[16] 2015	USA	COPD patients (n = 44)	Consecutive patients with COPD (37% on LTOT)	Age 67, 54% male	AHI ≥5	65.9%
Hu et al,[106] 2020	China	COPD patients (n = 968)	Consecutive outpatients with COPD	Age 65, 85% male	AHI ≥5	68.20%
Zhu et al,[107] 2020	China	COPD patients (n = 766)	Consecutive patients with COPD	Age 65, 85% male	AHI ≥5	68.90%
Zhao et al,[108] 2022	China	COPD patients (n = 252)	Consecutive patients with COPD	Age 64, 69% male	AHI ≥5	71.0%
Xiong et al,[64] 2019	China	COPD patients (n = 431)	Consecutive patients with COPD	Age 67, 90% male	AHI ≥5	77.70%

Abbreviations: AHI, apnea–hypopnea index; COPD, chronic obstructive pulmonary disease; LTOT, long-term oxygen therapy; OSA, obstructive pulmonary disease; OVS, overlap syndrome.
Note: Sleep lab, Consecutive patients undergoing in-laboratory polysomnography.

generate greater diaphragm muscle activity for a given minute ventilation compared to healthy subjects.[30] During sleep, there is increased mechanical load on the diaphragm and in healthy subjects, this is accompanied by an increase in diaphragmatic muscle activity to maintain minute ventilation.[31] In contrast, diaphragm activity drops significantly during sleep in patients with COPD—by 31% during non-REM sleep and 49% during REM sleep—resulting in significant nocturnal hypoventilation.[32] The combined effects of these changes mean that sleep represents a period of extreme vulnerability for respiratory compromise in patients with COPD.

The combined effects of COPD and OSA on nocturnal hypoxia are thought to drive some of the complications associated with OVS.[33] The pattern of oxygen desaturation in patients with OSA typically demonstrates repetitive oxygen desaturation with return of oxygen saturation to baseline levels following termination of each respiratory event (**Fig. 1**). In patients with COPD, oxygen desaturation tends to occur during REM sleep due to muscle atonia and it can be sustained during this period. Patients with OVS experience repetitive oxygen desaturation but the degree of hypoxia may be more profound due to the presence of baseline hypoxia, which places them on the steeper slope of the oxygen–hemoglobin desaturation curve. The effects of chronic hypoxia

on pulmonary hemodynamics may explain why patients with OVS appear to have increased risk of pulmonary hypertension (PH) compared to patients with COPD or OSA alone.[9] Using cardiac MRI, Sharma and colleagues demonstrated that patients with OVS also have higher right ventricular (RV) mass and RV remodeling compared to patients with COPD alone and this correlated with the degree of nocturnal oxygen desaturation.[34]

OVERLAP SYNDROME AND CARDIOVASCULAR DISEASE

It is well documented that patients with COPD and patients with OSA have an increased prevalence of comorbid CVD.[35–41] In patients with COPD, the direct effects of smoking resulting in release of inflammatory mediators and the development of atherosclerosis, while oxidative stress due to chronic hypoxia and endothelial dysfunction also mediate some of this risk (**Fig. 2**).[42–44] There is also evidence of ongoing systemic inflammation from COPD itself even after smoking cessation, which also contributes to the risk of cardiovascular comorbidity.[45] In patients with OSA, sleep fragmentation, repetitive hypoxia, and endothelial dysfunction are thought to further contribute to increased cardiovascular risk.[39,46,47] These effects are likely additive in patients with OVS, leading to high rates of cardiovascular morbidity and

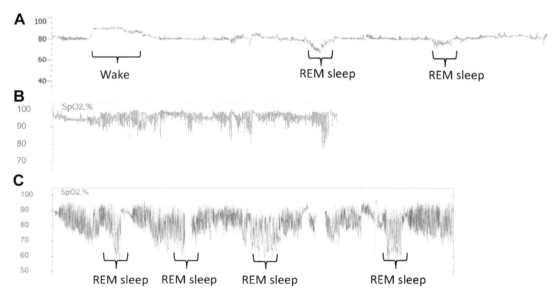

Fig. 1. Patterns of oxygen desaturation in patients with COPD (*A*), OSA (*B*), and OVS (*C*). In (*A*), oxygen saturation is 90% when the patient is awake but remains persistently reduced at 80% during sleep with periods of sustained desaturation during REM sleep. In (*B*), repetitive oxygen desaturation occurs, however, quickly returns to baseline in between oxygen desaturation episodes. In (*C*), repetitive and severe oxygen desaturation occurs with prolonged desaturation during REM sleep. COPD, chronic obstructive pulmonary disease; OSA, obstructive sleep apnea; OVS, overlap syndrome; REM, rapid eye movement.

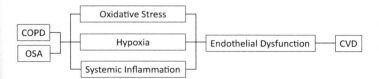

Fig. 2. Mechanism of cardiovascular disease in overlap syndrome. COPD, chronic obstructive pulmonary disease; OSA, obstructive sleep apnea; CVD, cardiovascular disease.

poor long-term outcomes. Tang and colleagues compared serum levels of brain natriuretic peptide (BNP) and cardiac troponins between patients with OVS, COPD, and OSA alone.[48] Both of these markers have demonstrated consistent associations with mortality in patients with heart failure and ischemic heart disease (IHD).[49–52] They found that patients with OVS had higher serum levels of BNP compared to patients with OSA alone; however, there were no differences in troponin levels between the 3 groups. Patients with OVS also have higher concentrations of inflammatory biomarkers including neutrophils, C-reactive protein, tumor necrosis factor-alpha, interleukin (IL)-6, and IL-8 compared to patients with COPD alone.[53–55] Furthermore, treatment of OSA with CPAP reduces both serum and airway markers of inflammation, although the impact of CPAP withdrawal models in OSA has provided some inconsistent results, with CPAP withdrawal not producing increases in markers of endothelial dysfunction, despite the return of OSA.[53,56]

There are numerous observational studies demonstrating an association between OVS and CVD including hypertension, IHD, atrial fibrillation, and PH.[8–10,57,58] A systematic review and meta-analysis reported that patients with OVS have a higher prevalence of systemic hypertension and PH compared to patients with COPD or OSA alone.[9] A subsequent meta-analysis excluded patients without spirometry-confirmed COPD and revealed a prevalence of IHD and hypertension in patients with OVS of 36% and 58%, respectively.[10] OVS was associated with a higher risk of hypertension compared to patients with COPD without OSA (odds ratio [OR] 1.68, 95% confidence interval [CI]: 1.21–2.35) and a higher risk of peripheral vascular disease compared to patients with OSA but without COPD (OR 3.3, 95% CI: 2.66–4.10). When patients with OVS are matched by age, sex, BMI, and AHI to patients with OSA but without COPD, there is more severe nocturnal hypoxemia and higher cardiovascular comorbidity, in particular heart failure and hypertension.[59] The link between sustained nocturnal hypoxia, independent of intermittent desaturation, driving cardiovascular comorbidity is also seen in patients with obesity hypoventilation syndrome, supporting this as a causative mechanism.[60] Notably, these data were derived from observational or non-randomized trials, with no randomized

controlled trials (RCTs) available in these analyses. In a prospective observational study, Machado and colleagues followed up 95 patients with COPD on long-term oxygen therapy and comorbid OSA over a median period of 41 months and found a mortality rate of 41%.[6] A significant proportion of the deaths (31%) were attributed to CVD. Marin and colleagues conducted a longer-term study with a median follow-up period of 9.5 years and found a similar mortality rate (37%) and proportion of death due to CVD (30%).[7]

OVERLAP SYNDROME AND RISK OF EXACERBATIONS

Patients with OVS have a greater than 3 fold risk of 30 day and 6 month hospital readmission for COPD exacerbations compared to patients with COPD alone, and the risk appears to be correlated with AHI.[61] In a prospective observational study, patients with OVS who were not treated with CPAP had a 1.7 times increased risk of hospitalization due to a COPD exacerbation compared to patients with COPD alone (95% CI 1.21–2.38).[7] A large retrospective cohort study examined clinical outcomes in 22,612 patients with OVS admitted to hospital with an acute exacerbation of COPD using State Inpatient Databases from 7 US states.[62] Patients with OVS were more likely to require noninvasive ventilation (NIV; OR 2.78, 95% CI 2.63–2.95) and had longer lengths of hospital stay (OR 1.19, 95% CI 1.15–1.23) compared to patients with COPD alone.

DIAGNOSIS

COPD and OSA are both very common respiratory conditions; however, there are some challenges in diagnosing OVS. Risk factors that may be associated with OSA such as age, gender, neck circumference, and Epworth Sleepiness Score may not apply to patients with OVS.[15,63] A large cross-sectional study including 46,786 patients with moderate-to-severe OSA and 2,098 patients with OVS, revealed that patients with OVS were less likely to report snoring, morning headaches, or subjective daytime sleepiness compared to patients with OSA alone.[58] BMI has been shown to correlate with the risk of OSA in patients with COPD[17,63] and the presence of CVD may also be a useful guide.[8–10,57,58] In one prospective observational study, the odds of comorbid OSA was 3.94 (95% CI 1.09–15.51) and 5.06 (95% CI 1.26–23.66) for BMI greater than 25 kg/m^2 and the presence of CVD respectively.[63] The use of BMI as a predictor for OVS was also supported in a recent cross-sectional study that demonstrated that the risk of OSA increases by 2.5 fold for every 1 kg/m^2 increase in BMI in patients with COPD.[54] Notwithstanding the differences in risk factors and reported symptoms, the use of screening tools such as the STOP-BANG questionnaire shows acceptable validity for use in identifying patients at higher risk of OSA in those with COPD.[64]

The diagnostic uncertainty of OVS is highlighted by inconsistencies in recommendations between guidelines produced by the American Thoracic Society and European Respiratory Society regarding whether sleep studies should be performed in patients with COPD and chronic hypercapnic respiratory failure.[65,66] Although no recommendation for PSG is made by the European Respiratory Society, the American Thoracic Society recommends that all patients with COPD and chronic hypercapnic respiratory failure should be screened for OSA prior to commencement of NIV.[65] While the guideline panel recognized that there may be some burdens associated with sleep testing in this population, they judged that where OSA was thought to be present, confirmatory testing with a sleep study could influence the type of PAP therapy prescribed (CPAP vs NIV) or aid in improving NIV titration. No recommendations around the level of sleep study were provided. In patients with COPD in whom a sleep study is felt indicated, the American Academy of Sleep Medicine recommends in-laboratory PSG rather than ambulatory sleep studies.[67] Other screening tools such as overnight oximetry may not be helpful in patients with COPD as these patients may demonstrate nocturnal desaturation due to reasons other than upper airway obstruction. However, there are data from a small study suggesting that the WatchPAT device (Itamar Medical Ltd, Cesarea, Israel) may have acceptable diagnostic accuracy to identify OSA in patients with COPD (sensitivity/specificity of 96%/55%, 92%/65%, and 89%/96% at an AHI cut-off of ≥5, ≥15, and ≥30, respectively) offering a more practical alternative to in-laboratory PSG.[29,68]

TREATMENT

There is little published guidance on treatment strategies for patients with OVS and a paucity of RCTs that assess the impact of treatment on clinical outcomes. Furthermore, there is lack of consensus on how to define OVS.[8–10] In contrast, the diagnosis and severity of COPD and OSA as separate entities are very well established and there are clear treatment guidelines for both conditions.[69,70] In general, the management of OVS comprises the relevant sections on guidance for COPD or OSA separately. It is also important to recognize that patients with OVS have a high prevalence of CVD and this needs to be managed accordingly. This section will focus on positive airway pressure (PAP) therapy as this has the most evidence in the treatment of OVS.

Although patients with OVS may not report the same degree of daytime symptoms compared to patients with OSA alone, treatment with CPAP appears to improve subjective scores of sleepiness, fatigue, and depression, regardless of baseline symptoms.[71] There are also a number of observational studies suggesting that CPAP may reduce the risk of COPD exacerbations and improve survival in patients with OVS.[6,7,72,73] In one study evaluating stable patients in the community, treatment with CPAP improved survival and reduced the risk of COPD exacerbations in patients with OVS compared to untreated or noncompliant patients.[7] Another observational study, again using a comparator group of noncompliant or untreated patients, assessed survival in patients with OSA and moderate-to-severe COPD requiring long-term oxygen therapy.[6] The 5 year survival rate was 71% (95% CI 53%–83%) in patients treated with CPAP and 26% (95% CI 12%–43%) in patients who were not treated. The use of a "control" group consisting of patients who refused or were nonadherent to treatment, raises the possibility of biases such as the "healthy user effect."[74] It is well established that patients who exhibit positive health behaviors, such as treatment adherence, have improved outcomes likely mediated by other associated positive health behaviors, making the estimation of a genuine treatment effect from these studies difficult.[75] Another retrospective study demonstrated an association between CPAP usage and survival in patients with OVS.[73] In a post hoc analysis, greater hours of CPAP usage was associated with a reduction in mortality (hazard ratio 0.71, 95% CI 0.55–0.90). The importance of CPAP adherence in patients with OVS was reinforced in another recent observational study where good adherence was defined as CPAP usage of more than 4 hours per night on more than 70% of nights. Patients who demonstrated poor CPAP adherence had 0.362 more COPD exacerbations than patients with good adherence (95% CI 0.075–0.649).[76] A recent retrospective observational study linked a large US claims database with PAP usage data obtained by remote monitoring, compared health outcomes between patients with OVS who were compliant with PAP therapy and non-compliant patients.[72] They found that patients who were compliant with CPAP had significantly improved clinical outcomes as defined by reduced Emergency Department visits, hospitalization, and severe acute exacerbation frequency, and reduced health care costs compared to patients who were not compliant.

NIV is a well-established treatment for acute hypercapnic COPD[69,77,78] and clinical guidelines also support a role for NIV in stable COPD patients with chronic hypercapnia.[65,66,78,79] While most studies have demonstrated worse clinical outcomes in patients with OVS compared to patients with COPD alone, this may not hold true for patients once treated with long-term NIV. A large European study examined long-term survival of patients who were initiated on home NIV for chronic hypercapnic respiratory failure due to a variety of causes.[80] In this cohort, patients with OVS had longer survival compared to patients with COPD alone, with a median survival of 6.6 and 2.7 years, respectively. The reason for this discordancy is unclear; however, patients with COPD alone in this cohort had likely reached the end stage of their disease and would therefore be expected to have a higher mortality. Although patients with OVS on long-term NIV had lower mortality, the patient groups were not necessarily comparable and prospective studies will be required to clarify the role of NIV in patients with OVS.

One of the first published randomized controlled trials in patients with OVS revealed that NIV was superior to CPAP in reducing arterial carbon dioxide ($Paco_2$; 9.4 mm Hg, 95% CI 4.3–15 mm Hg).[81] As this was only a pilot study with 32 participants and a short follow-up period of 3 months, clinical outcomes such as health care utilization and mortality were unable to be assessed. Recent clinical trials in patients with stable hypercapnic COPD have demonstrated a survival benefit when NIV was set with the goal of reducing $Paco_2$ maximally.[82,83] Such an approach may also produce more favorable results in patients with OVS. These findings provide some insights for future clinical trials comparing NIV with CPAP in patients with OVS and chronic hypercapnia.

Finally, there may be a role for PAP therapy to improve exercise capacity in patients with OVS. Reduced physical activity has been associated with worse clinical outcomes in patients with COPD including higher risk of acute exacerbations, hospitalizations and death.[84,85] Patients with COPD and patients with OSA have reduced physical activity compared to their healthy peers[86,87] and there is evidence that patients with OVS may have even lower levels of physical activity.[88] Fitzgibbons and colleagues used pedometers to objectively measure physical activity and found that patients with OVS walked on average 672 fewer steps per day (95% CI -1317–28, $P = .41$) compared to patients with COPD alone.[88] CPAP has been shown to improve exercise performance in patients with OSA, even in the absence of any changes in BMI.[89,90] Two separate observational studies utilized cardiopulmonary exercise testing and found that maximal workload and peak oxygen consumption increased following 2 months of CPAP therapy in patients with OSA. One study has evaluated the use of CPAP therapy on exercise capacity in patients with OVS and patients with COPD alone.[91] After only 2 nights of CPAP therapy, patients with OVS achieved a significantly greater change in walking distance on the incremental shuttle walking test compared to patients with COPD (62.3 ± 24.9 m vs 15.1 ± 33.6 m, respectively). There were several limitations to this study including its observational design, small sample size, and poor compliance rate with only 45% of OVS participants using CPAP for at least 4 hours per night. Larger randomized trials will be required to clarify the impact of CPAP on exercise in patients with OVS, while the utility of NIV in this regard remains to be explored.

SUMMARY

COPD–OSA OVS is common and confers significant increased cardiovascular morbidity and exacerbation risk. The driver of cardiovascular morbidity requires further work to elucidate the mechanism but appears in part driven by hypoxia and systemic inflammation. The ability of PAP therapy to attenuate these risks remains to be proven but it does appear to improve sleep symptoms in patients with OVS. There are a lack of guidelines on the management of OVS due to the paucity of good quality randomized controlled trials in this area and this should be the focus of future work. In particular, the ability of PAP therapy to reduce COPD exacerbations, hospitalization, and death, and whether there are clinically meaningful differences between CPAP or NIV in the management of patients with OVS needs further investigation.

DISCLOSURE

Dr P.B. Murphy reported receiving reimbursement for expenses for travel to conferences and lecture fees from Philips Respironics, ResMed, Fisher & Paykel, Chiesi, Genzyme and Breas Medical.

REFERENCES

1. Flenley DC. Sleep in chronic obstructive lung disease. Clin Chest Med 1985;6(4):651–61.
2. Malhotra A, Schwartz AR, Schneider H, et al. Research priorities in pathophysiology for sleep-disordered breathing in patients with chronic obstructive pulmonary disease. An official American thoracic society research statement. Am J Respir Crit Care Med 2018;197(3):289–99.
3. Lurie A, Roche N. Obstructive sleep apnea in patients with chronic obstructive pulmonary disease: facts and perspectives. COPD 2021;18(6):700–12.
4. Agustí A, Hogg JC. Update on the pathogenesis of chronic obstructive pulmonary disease. N Engl J Med 2019;381(13):1248–56.
5. Veasey SC, Rosen IM. Obstructive sleep apnea in adults. N Engl J Med 2019;380(15):1442–9.
6. Machado M-CL, Vollmer WM, Togeiro SM, et al. CPAP and survival in moderate-to-severe obstructive sleep apnoea syndrome and hypoxaemic COPD. Eur Respir J 2010;35(1):132–7.
7. Marin JM, Soriano JB, Carrizo SJ, et al. Outcomes in patients with chronic obstructive pulmonary disease and obstructive sleep apnea: the overlap syndrome. Am J Respir Crit Care Med 2010;182(3):325–31.
8. Shawon MS, Perret JL, Senaratna CV, et al. Current evidence on prevalence and clinical outcomes of co-morbid obstructive sleep apnea and chronic obstructive pulmonary disease: a systematic review. Sleep Med Rev 2017;32:58–68.
9. Xu J, Wei Z, Wang X, et al. The risk of cardiovascular and cerebrovascular disease in overlap syndrome: a meta-analysis. J Clin Sleep Med 2020;16(7):1199–207.
10. Shah AJ, Quek E, Alqahtani JS, et al. Cardiovascular outcomes in patients with COPD-OSA overlap syndrome: a systematic review and meta-analysis. Sleep Med Rev 2022;63:101627.
11. Brennan M, McDonnell MJ, Walsh SM, et al. Review of the prevalence, pathogenesis and management of OSA-COPD overlap. Sleep Breath 2022;26(4):1551–60.
12. Czerwaty K, Dżaman K, Sobczyk KM, et al. The overlap syndrome of obstructive sleep apnea and chronic obstructive pulmonary disease: a systematic review. Biomedicines 2022;11(1):16.
13. Turcani P, Skrickova J, Pavlik T, et al. The prevalence of obstructive sleep apnea in patients hospitalized for COPD exacerbation. Biomed Pap Med Fac Univ Palacky Olomouc Czech Repub 2015;159(3):422–8.
14. Venkateswaran S, Tee A. Overlap syndrome between chronic obstructive pulmonary disease and obstructive sleep apnoea in a Southeast Asian teaching hospital. Singapore Med J 2014;55(9):488–92.
15. Sanders MH, Newman AB, Haggerty CL, et al. Sleep and sleep-disordered breathing in adults with predominantly mild obstructive airway disease. Am J Respir Crit Care Med 2003;167(1):7–14.
16. Soler X, Gaio E, Powell FL, et al. High prevalence of obstructive sleep apnea in patients with moderate to severe chronic obstructive pulmonary disease. Ann Am Thorac Soc 2015;12(8):1219–25.
17. Steveling EH, Clarenbach CF, Miedinger D, et al. Predictors of the overlap syndrome and its association with comorbidities in patients with chronic obstructive pulmonary disease. Respiration 2014;88(6):451–7.
18. Owens RL, Malhotra A, Eckert DJ, et al. The influence of end-expiratory lung volume on measurements of pharyngeal collapsibility. J Appl Physiol 2010;108(2):445–51.
19. Biselli P, Grossman PR, Kirkness JP, et al. The effect of increased lung volume in chronic obstructive pulmonary disease on upper airway obstruction during sleep. J Appl Physiol 2015;119(3):266–71.
20. Kairaitis K, Byth K, Parikh R, et al. Tracheal traction effects on upper airway patency in rabbits: the role of tissue pressure. Sleep 2007;30(2):179–86.
21. Krachman SL, Tiwari R, Vega ME, et al. Effect of emphysema severity on the apnea-hypopnea index in smokers with obstructive sleep apnea. Ann Am Thorac Soc 2016;13(7):1129–35.
22. Douglas NJ, White DP, Pickett CK, et al. Respiration during sleep in normal man. Thorax 1982;37(11):840–4.
23. Stradling JR, Chadwick GA, Frew AJ. Changes in ventilation and its components in normal subjects during sleep. Thorax 1985;40(5):364–70.
24. Hudgel DW, Devadatta P. Decrease in functional residual capacity during sleep in normal humans. J Appl Physiol Respir Environ Exerc Physiol 1984;57(5):1319–22.
25. Douglas NJ, White DP, Weil JV, et al. Hypoxic ventilatory response decreases during sleep in normal men. Am Rev Respir Dis 1982;125(3):286–9.
26. Berthon-Jones M, Sullivan CE. Ventilatory and arousal responses to hypoxia in sleeping humans. Am Rev Respir Dis 1982;125(6):632–9.
27. Midgren B, Hansson L. Changes in transcutaneous PCO2 with sleep in normal subjects and in patients with chronic respiratory diseases. Eur J Respir Dis 1987;71(5):388–94.
28. Wade OL. Movements of the thoracic cage and diaphragm in respiration. J Physiol 1954;124(2):193–212.
29. McNicholas WT. COPD-OSA overlap syndrome: evolving evidence regarding epidemiology, clinical

consequences, and management. Chest 2017; 152(6):1318–26.

30. Jolley CJ, Luo YM, Steier J, et al. Neural respiratory drive in healthy subjects and in COPD. Eur Respir J 2009;33(2):289–97.

31. Tabachnik E, Muller NL, Bryan AC, et al. Changes in ventilation and chest wall mechanics during sleep in normal adolescents. J Appl Physiol Respir Environ Exerc Physiol 1981;51(3):557–64.

32. Luo YM, He BT, Wu YX, et al. Neural respiratory drive and ventilation in patients with chronic obstructive pulmonary disease during sleep. Am J Respir Crit Care Med 2014;190(2):227–9.

33. Owens RL, Malhotra A. Sleep-disordered breathing and COPD: the overlap syndrome. Respir Care 2010;55(10):1333–44. discussion 1344-1336.

34. Sharma B, Neilan TG, Kwong RY, et al. Evaluation of right ventricular remodeling using cardiac magnetic resonance imaging in co-existent chronic obstructive pulmonary disease and obstructive sleep apnea. COPD 2013;10(1):4–10.

35. Morgan AD, Zakeri R, Quint JK. Defining the relationship between COPD and CVD: what are the implications for clinical practice? Ther Adv Respir Dis 2018;12. 1753465817750524.

36. Rabe KF, Hurst JR, Suissa S. Cardiovascular disease and COPD: dangerous liaisons? Eur Respir Rev 2018;27(149):180057.

37. Yacoub M, Youssef I, Salifu MO, et al. Cardiovascular disease risk in obstructive sleep apnea: an update. J Sleep Disord Ther 2018;7(1):283.

38. McNicholas WT, Bonsignore MR. B26 tMCoECA. Sleep apnoea as an independent risk factor for cardiovascular disease: current evidence, basic mechanisms and research priorities. Eur Respir J 2007;29(1):156–78.

39. Bradley TD, Floras JS. Obstructive sleep apnoea and its cardiovascular consequences. Lancet 2009;373(9657):82–93.

40. Feary JR, Rodrigues LC, Smith CJ, et al. Prevalence of major comorbidities in subjects with COPD and incidence of myocardial infarction and stroke: a comprehensive analysis using data from primary care. Thorax 2010;65(11):956–62.

41. Young T, Finn L, Peppard PE, et al. Sleep disordered breathing and mortality: eighteen-year follow-up of the Wisconsin sleep cohort. Sleep 2008;31(8):1071–8.

42. Drakopoulou M, Toutouzas K, Michelongona A, et al. Vulnerable plaque and inflammation: potential clinical strategies. Curr Pharmaceut Des 2011; 17(37):4190–209.

43. Vivodtzev I, Tamisier R, Baguet JP, et al. Arterial stiffness in COPD. Chest 2014;145(4):861–75.

44. Sin DD, Man SF. Why are patients with chronic obstructive pulmonary disease at increased risk of cardiovascular diseases? The potential role of systemic inflammation in chronic obstructive pulmonary disease. Circulation 2003;107(11):1514–9.

45. Sin DD, Anthonisen NR, Soriano JB, et al. Mortality in COPD: role of comorbidities. Eur Respir J 2006; 28(6):1245–57.

46. Smith ML, Niedermaier ON, Hardy SM, et al. Role of hypoxemia in sleep apnea-induced sympathoexcitation. J Auton Nerv Syst 1996;56(3):184–90.

47. Shamsuzzaman ASM, Winnicki M, Lanfranchi P, et al. Elevated C-reactive protein in patients with obstructive sleep apnea. Circulation 2002; 105(21):2462–4.

48. Tang M, Wang Y, Wang M, et al. Risk for cardiovascular disease and one-year mortality in patients with chronic obstructive pulmonary disease and obstructive sleep apnea syndrome overlap syndrome. Front Pharmacol 2021;12:767982.

49. York MK, Gupta DK, Reynolds CF, et al. B-type natriuretic peptide levels and mortality in patients with and without heart failure. J Am Coll Cardiol 2018;71(19):2079–88.

50. Berger R, Huelsman M, Strecker K, et al. B-type natriuretic peptide predicts sudden death in patients with chronic heart failure. Circulation 2002; 105(20):2392–7.

51. Doust JA, Pietrzak E, Dobson A, et al. How well does B-type natriuretic peptide predict death and cardiac events in patients with heart failure: systematic review. BMJ 2005;330(7492):625.

52. Everett BM, Brooks MM, Vlachos HE, et al, BARI 2D Study Group. Troponin and cardiac events in stable ischemic heart disease and diabetes. N Engl J Med 2015;373(7):610–20.

53. Wang Y, Hu K, Liu K, et al. Obstructive sleep apnea exacerbates airway inflammation in patients with chronic obstructive pulmonary disease. Sleep Med 2015;16(9):1123–30.

54. Zhou W, Li CL, Cao J, et al. Metabolic syndrome prevalence in patients with obstructive sleep apnea syndrome and chronic obstructive pulmonary disease: relationship with systemic inflammation. Clin Respir J 2020;14(12):1159–65.

55. Fitzgibbons C, Goldstein R, Gottlieb DJ, et al. Overlap syndrome of COPD and osa: metabolic risk factors and systemic inflammation, Sleep, 40, 2017, ATS conference, 195. American journal of respiratory and critical care medicine conference: American thoracic society international conference.

56. Turnbull CD, Rossi VA, Santer P, et al. Effect of OSA on hypoxic and inflammatory markers during CPAP withdrawal: further evidence from three randomized control trials. Respirology 2017;22(4):793–9.

57. Kendzerska T, Leung RS, Aaron SD, et al. Cardiovascular outcomes and all-cause mortality in patients with obstructive sleep apnea and chronic obstructive pulmonary disease (overlap syndrome). Ann Am Thorac Soc 2019;16(1):71–81.

58. Adle D, Bailly S, Benmerad M, et al. Clinical presentation and comorbidities of obstructive sleep apnea-COPD overlap syndrome. PLoS One 2020; 15(7):e0235331.

59. van Zeller M, Basoglu OK, Verbraecken J, et al. Sleep and cardiometabolic comorbidities in the obstructive sleep apnoea-COPD overlap syndrome: data from the European Sleep Apnoea Database. ERJ Open Res 2023;9(3):00676-2022.

60. Baumert M, Immanuel SA, Stone KL, et al. Composition of nocturnal hypoxaemic burden and its prognostic value for cardiovascular mortality in older community-dwelling men. Eur Heart J 2020; 41(4):533-41.

61. Naranjo M, Willes L, Prillaman BA, et al. Undiagnosed OSA may significantly affect outcomes in adults admitted for COPD in an inner-city hospital. Chest 2020;158(3):1198-207.

62. Hirayama A, Goto T, Faridi MK, et al. Association of obstructive sleep apnoea with acute severity of chronic obstructive pulmonary disease exacerbation: a population-based study. Intern Med J 2018;48(9):1150-3.

63. Soler X, Liao SY, Marin JM, et al. Age, gender, neck circumference, and Epworth sleepiness scale do not predict obstructive sleep apnea (OSA) in moderate to severe chronic obstructive pulmonary disease (COPD): the challenge to predict OSA in advanced COPD. PLoS One 2017; 12(5):e0177289.

64. Xiong M, Hu W, Dong M, et al. The screening value of ESS, SACS, BQ, and SBQ on obstructive sleep apnea in patients with chronic obstructive pulmonary disease. Int J Chronic Obstr Pulm Dis 2019; 14:2497-505.

65. Macrea M, Oczkowski S, Rochwerg B, et al. Long-term noninvasive ventilation in chronic stable hypercapnic chronic obstructive pulmonary disease. An official American thoracic society clinical practice guideline. Am J Respir Crit Care Med 2020; 202(4):e74-87.

66. Ergan B, Oczkowski S, Rochwerg B, et al. European Respiratory Society guidelines on long-term home non-invasive ventilation for management of COPD. Eur Respir J 2019;54(3):1901003.

67. Kapur VK, Auckley DH, Chowdhuri S, et al. Clinical practice guideline for diagnostic testing for adult obstructive sleep apnea: an American Academy of sleep medicine clinical practice guideline. J Clin Sleep Med 2017;13(03):479-504.

68. Jen R, Orr JE, Li Y, et al. Accuracy of WatchPAT for the diagnosis of obstructive sleep apnea in patients with chronic obstructive pulmonary disease. COPD 2020;17(1):34-9.

69. Global Initiative for Chronic Obstructive Lung Disease, Global strategy for prevention, diagnosis and management of COPD: 2023 report, 2023, Global Initiative for Chronic Obstructive Lung Disease, Available at: https://goldcopd.org/2023-gold-report-2/. Accessed November 18, 2023.

70. Patil SP, Ayappa IA, Caples SM, et al. Treatment of adult obstructive sleep apnea with positive airway pressure: an American Academy of sleep medicine clinical practice guideline. J Clin Sleep Med 2019; 15(02):335-43.

71. Adler D, Bailly S, Soccal PM, et al. Symptomatic response to CPAP in obstructive sleep apnea versus COPD- obstructive sleep apnea overlap syndrome: insights from a large national registry. PLoS One 2021;16(8):e0256230.

72. Sterling KL, Pépin JL, Linde-Zwirble W, et al. Impact of positive airway pressure therapy adherence on outcomes in patients with obstructive sleep apnea and chronic obstructive pulmonary disease. Am J Respir Crit Care Med 2022;206(2): 197-205.

73. Stanchina ML, Welicky LM, Donat W, et al. Impact of CPAP use and age on mortality in patients with combined COPD and obstructive sleep apnea: the overlap syndrome. J Clin Sleep Med 2013; 9(8):767-72.

74. Granger BB, Swedberg K, Ekman I, et al. Adherence to candesartan and placebo and outcomes in chronic heart failure in the CHARM programme: double-blind, randomised, controlled clinical trial. Lancet 2005;366(9502):2005-11.

75. Donovan LM, Patel SR. The challenges of estimating causal effects of continuous positive airway pressure therapy from observational data. Am J Respir Crit Care Med 2022;206(12):1570-1.

76. Voulgaris A, Archontogeorgis K, Anevlavis S, et al. Effect of compliance to continuous positive airway pressure on exacerbations, lung function and symptoms in patients with chronic obstructive pulmonary disease and obstructive sleep apnea (overlap syndrome). Clin Respir J 2023;17(3): 165-75.

77. Rochwerg B, Brochard L, Elliott MW, et al. Official ERS/ATS clinical practice guidelines: noninvasive ventilation for acute respiratory failure. Eur Respir J 2017;50(2):1602426.

78. British Thoracic Society Standards of Care Committee. Non-invasive ventilation in acute respiratory failure. Thorax 2002;57(3):192.

79. Raveling T, Vonk J, Struik FM, et al. Chronic non-invasive ventilation for chronic obstructive pulmonary disease. Cochrane Database Syst Rev 2021; 8(8):CD002878.

80. Patout M, Lhuillier E, Kaltsakas G, et al. Long-term survival following initiation of home non-invasive ventilation: a European study. Thorax 2020;75(11): 965-73.

81. Zheng Y, Yee BJ, Wong K, et al. A pilot randomized trial comparing CPAP vs bilevel PAP spontaneous

mode in the treatment of hypoventilation disorder in patients with obesity and obstructive airway disease. J Clin Sleep Med 2022;18(1):99–107.

82. Murphy PB, Rehal S, Arbane G, et al. Effect of home noninvasive ventilation with oxygen therapy vs oxygen therapy alone on hospital readmission or death after an acute COPD exacerbation: a randomized clinical trial. JAMA 2017;317(21): 2177–86.

83. Köhnlein T, Windisch W, Köhler D, et al. Non-invasive positive pressure ventilation for the treatment of severe stable chronic obstructive pulmonary disease: a prospective, multicentre, randomised, controlled clinical trial. Lancet Respir Med 2014; 2(9):698–705.

84. Waschki B, Kirsten A, Holz O, et al. Physical activity is the strongest predictor of all-cause mortality in patients with COPD: a prospective cohort study. Chest 2011;140(2):331–42.

85. Garcia-Aymerich J, Lange P, Benet M, et al. Regular physical activity reduces hospital admission and mortality in chronic obstructive pulmonary disease: a populaton based cohort study. Thorax 2006;61(9):772–8.

86. Pitta F, Troosters T, Spruit MA, et al. Characteristics of physical activities in daily life in chronic obstructive pulmonary disease. Am J Respir Crit Care Med 2005;171(9):972–7.

87. Hargens TA, Martin RA, Strosnider CL, et al. Obstructive sleep apnea negatively impacts objectively measured physical activity. Sleep Breath 2019;23(2):447–54.

88. Fitzgibbons CM, Goldstein RL, Gottlieb DJ, et al. Physical activity in overlap syndrome of COPD and obstructive sleep apnea: relationship with markers of systemic inflammation. J Clin Sleep Med 2019;15(7):973–8.

89. Quadri F, Boni E, Pini L, et al. Exercise tolerance in obstructive sleep apnea-hypopnea (OSAH), before and after CPAP treatment: effects of autonomic dysfunction improvement. Respir Physiol Neurobiol 2017;236:51–6.

90. Lin CC, Lin CK, Wu KM, et al. Effect of treatment by nasal CPAP on cardiopulmonary exercise test in obstructive sleep apnea syndrome. Lung 2004; 182:199–212.

91. Wang TY, Lo YL, Lee KY, et al. Nocturnal CPAP improves walking capacity in COPD patients with obstructive sleep apnoea. Respir Res 2013;14(1): 66.

92. Bednarek M, Plywaczewski R, Jonczak L, Zielinski J. There is no relationship between chronic obstructive pulmonary disease and obstructive sleep apnea syndrome: a population study. Respiration 2005;72(2):142–9.

93. Chaouat A, Weitzenblum E, Krieger J, et al. Association of chronic obstructive pulmonary disease and sleep apnea syndrome. Am J Respir Crit Care Med 1995;151(1):82–6.

94. Shiina K, Tomiyama H, Takata Y, et al. Overlap syndrome: additive effects of COPD on the cardiovascular damages in patients with OSA. Respir Med 2012;106(9):1335–41.

95. Rizzi M, Palma P, Andreoli A, et al. Prevalence and clinical feature of the "overlap syndrome", obstructive sleep apnea (OSA) and chronic obstructive pulmonary disease (COPD), in OSA population. Sleep Breath 1997;2:68–72.

96. López-Acevedo MN, Torres-Palacios A, Elena Ocasio-Tascón M, et al. Overlap syndrome: an indication for sleep studies? : A pilot study. Sleep Breath 2009;13(4):409–13.

97. Perimenis P, Karkoulias K, Konstantinopoulos A, et al. The impact of long-term conventional treatment for overlap syndrome (obstructive sleep apnea and chronic obstructive pulmonary disease) on concurrent erectile dysfunction. Respir Med 2007;101(2):210–6.

98. Zhang P, Chen B, Lou H, et al. Predictors and outcomes of obstructive sleep apnea in patients with chronic obstructive pulmonary disease in China. BMC Pulm Med 2022;22(1):16.

99. Zeng Z, Song Y, He X, et al. Obstructive Sleep Apnea is Associated with an Increased Prevalence of Polycythemia in Patients with Chronic Obstructive Pulmonary Disease. Int J Chron Obstruct Pulmon Dis 2022;17:195–204.

100. Wang Y, Li B, Li P, et al. Severe obstructive sleep apnea in patients with chronic obstructive pulmonary disease is associated with an increased prevalence of mild cognitive impairment. Sleep Med 2020;75:522–30.

101. Zhang XL, Dai HP, Zhang H, et al. Obstructive Sleep Apnea in Patients With Fibrotic Interstitial Lung Disease and COPD. J Clin Sleep Med 2019; 15(12):1807–15.

102. Zhang XL, Gao B, Han T, et al. Moderate-to-Severe Obstructive Sleep Apnea and Cognitive Function Impairment in Patients with COPD. Int J Chron Obstruct Pulmon Dis 2020;15:1813–22.

103. Clímaco DCS, Lustosa TC, Silva MVFP, et al. Sleep quality in COPD patients: correlation with disease severity and health status. J Bras Pneumol 2022; 48(3):e20210340.

104. Wu Q, Xie L, Li W, et al. Pulmonary Function Influences the Performance of Berlin Questionnaire, Modified Berlin Questionnaire, and STOP-Bang Score for Screening Obstructive Sleep Apnea in Subjects with Chronic Obstructive Pulmonary Disease. Int J Chron Obstruct Pulmon Dis 2020;15: 1207–16.

105. Yang X, Tang X, Cao Y, et al. The Bronchiectasis in COPD-OSA Overlap Syndrome Patients. Int J Chron Obstruct Pulmon Dis 2020;15:605–11.

106. Hu W, Zhao Z, Wu B, et al. Obstructive Sleep Apnea Increases the Prevalence of Hypertension in Patients with Chronic Obstructive Disease. COPD 2020;17(5):523–32.

107. Zhu J, Zhao Z, Nie Q, et al. Effect of lung function on the apnea-hypopnea index in patients with overlap syndrome: a multicenter cross-sectional study. Sleep Breath 2020;24(3):1059–66.

108. Zhao Z, Zhang D, Sun H, et al. Anxiety and depression in patients with chronic obstructive pulmonary disease and obstructive sleep apnea: the overlap syndrome. Sleep Breath 2022;26(4):1603–11.

Initiation of Chronic Non-invasive Ventilation

Marieke L. Duiverman, MD, PhD[a],*, Filipa Jesus, MD[a,b], Gerrie Bladder, RN[a], Peter J. Wijkstra, MD, PhD[a]

KEYWORDS

- Non-invasive ventilation • Home mechanical ventilation • Initiation • Monitoring • Telemonitoring
- Neuromuscular disease • Obesity hypoventilation syndrome
- Chronic obstructive pulmonary disease

KEY POINTS

- Before starting home non-invasive ventilation (NIV), patients need to be provided with appropriate information about the expected benefits (symptom reduction, survival benefit), potential difficulties, and side effects of NIV, while also being given time to process this information.
- The decision to start NIV is based on a combination of patient symptoms and objective evidence of sleep-related hypoventilation, with the urgency to start varying with the expected progression of the underlying disease.
- Appropriate setting of ventilator parameters requires a solid understanding of the pathophysiology of the patient's underlying disease process.
- NIV can be initiated in any comfortable, safe environment where sufficient monitoring of ventilator output and efficacy can be assured.

INTRODUCTION

Chronic nocturnal non-invasive ventilation (NIV) has been shown to be effective in patients with chronic respiratory failure due to sleep-related hypoventilation in a range of different underlying diseases, including neuromuscular diseases (NMD),[1–4] restrictive thoracic diseases (including obesity hypoventilation syndrome [OHS]),[5] and lung diseases (including chronic obstructive pulmonary disease [COPD]).[6,7] As patients often use NIV at home for years, optimal preparation and titration of NIV settings is necessary to achieve good adherence and maximize the benefits of therapy. However, the pathophysiology of different underlying diseases is variable, and thus titration of NIV should be tailored to this underlying pathophysiology. In this review, the authors discuss indications and provide practical guidance on initiation

(**Table 1**) and titration (**Table 2**; **Fig. 1**) of NIV in different diseases, as well as discussing monitoring during the titration period, including a focus on the location where NIV is initiated. As positive pressure ventilation is currently the mode of choice in the majority of home-ventilated patients, we will focus on this mode of ventilation.

INITIATION OF CHRONIC NON-INVASIVE VENTILATION IN NEUROMUSCULAR DISEASE

While NMD encompasses a wide variety of diseases, when respiratory failure develops the common pathophysiology is respiratory muscle weakness/dysfunction. The progression of respiratory muscle weakness and thus the urgency with which to start respiratory support and the prognosis of the different diseases varies among the different NMDs. Notwithstanding severe bulbar

a Department of Pulmonary Diseases/Home Mechanical Ventilation, University of Groningen, University Medical Center Groningen, Groningen, the Netherlands; b Pulmonology Department, Unidade Local de Saúde da Guarda EPE, Rainha D. Amélia, s/n 6301-857 Guarda, Portugal
* Corresponding author. University Medical Center Groningen. Department of Pulmonary Diseases/Home Mechanical Ventilation, home postal code AA62. Hanzeplein 1. 9700 RB, Groningen, the Netherlands.
E-mail address: m.l.duiverman@umcg.nl

Sleep Med Clin 19 (2024) 419–430
https://doi.org/10.1016/j.jsmc.2024.04.006

Table 1
Summary of issues to be considered before starting

	Before Starting Therapy	Choosing when to Start Treatment
Relevant for every patient	• Adequate information • Preferably time to consider the intervention • Patient's motivation and expectations • Consideration of feasibility, safety (circumstances) • Shared decision-making	
NMD	• Multidisciplinary care path • Family involvement • Prepare for the future (advanced care planning)	• Combination of symptoms, objective evidence of hypoventilation (including nocturnal monitoring) and expected progression of the disease • Regular follow-up
OHS	• Discuss the need for multidisciplinary treatment including lifestyle changes • Preferably a diagnostic sleep study to look for concomitant OSA	• CPAP or NIV? • Acute on chronic respiratory failure: likely require NIV in the acute setting • Consider switching to CPAP longer term with OHS/OSA
COPD	• Phenotype patients • Also consider other potential treatment options (look at treatable traits) • Prepare for the future (advanced care planning)	Persistent or chronic hypercapnia, that is, $Pa_{CO_2} > 6.0$ kPa (45 mm Hg) with symptoms of nocturnal hypoventilation

Abbreviations: COPD, chronic obstructive pulmonary disease; CPAP, continuous positive airway pressure; NMD, neuromuscular disease; NIV, non-invasive ventilation; OHS, obesity hypoventilation syndrome; OSA, obstructive sleep apnea.

weakness limiting the application of NIV in some patients, in most cases of NMD, NIV will be the therapy of first choice, often in combination with cough assist techniques.[8,9]

Before Commencing Non-invasive Ventilation

Before starting NIV, patients must receive appropriate information about the intervention and then in the context of being well informed, be allowed time to decide whether to proceed with NIV. This requires the patient to understand the expected gains (symptom reduction, survival benefit), the steps involved in establishing therapy, and potential side effects of NIV. In addition, feasibility, safety, and social circumstances should be carefully considered. In some diseases, the expected benefit is so great that it will almost always overrule any disadvantages,[10] especially in patients with progressive conditions such as rapidly progressive motor neuron disease (MND). However, in other cases the benefit may not outweigh the side effects or deleterious consequences on the patient's social circumstances (for instance, patients who have to relocate to a care facility to allow NIV to be safely provided).

The decision to start NIV should therefore always be a shared decision, preferably as part of specialized multidisciplinary care clinic, which also involves family and caregivers.[11,12] Prior to commencing NIV, it is preferable to discuss the possible trajectory that after starting nocturnal NIV, disease progression may lead to more extended daytime use of NIV, and, in a minority of patients, tracheostomy ventilation. This information should be provided at an early stage of the disease process, when the patient is still able to communicate and participate actively in their medical care. This allows patients and their families to make well-informed decisions about what they do or do not want, while also guiding action plans in the setting of an acute deterioration.[13]

Timing of Commencement of Non-invasive Ventilation

The decision to start NIV is based on a combination of patient symptoms and objective evidence of sleep-related hypoventilation within the context of the expected progression of the patient's underlying disease. In more slowly progressive diseases, such as myotonic dystrophy, starting NIV too early before the patient develops any symptoms, will potentially lead to noncompliance and unsuccessful therapy.[14,15] In patients with rapidly progressing NMD,

Table 2
Titration and ventilatory settings in different underlying pathophysiology

Underlying Pathophysiology	First Choice Mode	IPAP	EPAP	Tidal Volume	BURR	Trigger Sensitivity	Rise Time	Inspiration Time	Cycle Sensitivity
NMD	ST mode	Moderate (titrate for comfort and optimized gas exchange)	Low (minimum to ensure expiratory washout flow)	Sufficient to improve gas exchange	Moderate to high to ensure adequate minute ventilation	High to support weak respiratory muscle effort	Slow to ensure adequate time to achieve adequate distribution of ventilation	Long to ensure sufficient tidal volume (Ti/Tot: 1:2)	Low to ensure long inspiratory time
OHS	ST or volume-targeted pressure support ± auto-titrating EPAP	High (titrate for optimal gas exchange)	Often high to overcome upper airway resistance, titrate to eliminate upper airway obstruction and/or snoring	Sufficient to improve gas exchange	Moderate to ensure adequate minute ventilation	Medium to low	Slow to ensure gradual pressure rise for respiratory system with low compliance	Long to ensure sufficient tidal volume (Ti/Tot: 1:2)	Low to ensure long inspiratory time
COPD	ST mode	High enough to improve CO_2 exchange	High enough to counterbalance PEEP	Sufficient to improve gas exchange	Low to ensure sufficient expiratory time	Medium	Fast to ensure that IPAP is reached	Short to maximize expiratory time (Ti/Tot 1:4 or 1:5)	High to enable early cycling and long expiratory time

Abbreviations: BURR, back-up respiratory rate; CO_2, carbon dioxide; COPD, chronic obstructive pulmonary disease; EPAP, expiratory positive airway pressure; IPAP, inspiratory positive airway pressure; NMD, neuromuscular disease; OHS, obesity hypoventilation syndrome; PEEP, positive end-expiratory pressure; ST, spontaneous-timed; Ti/Ttot, inspiratory time/total time of one breath.

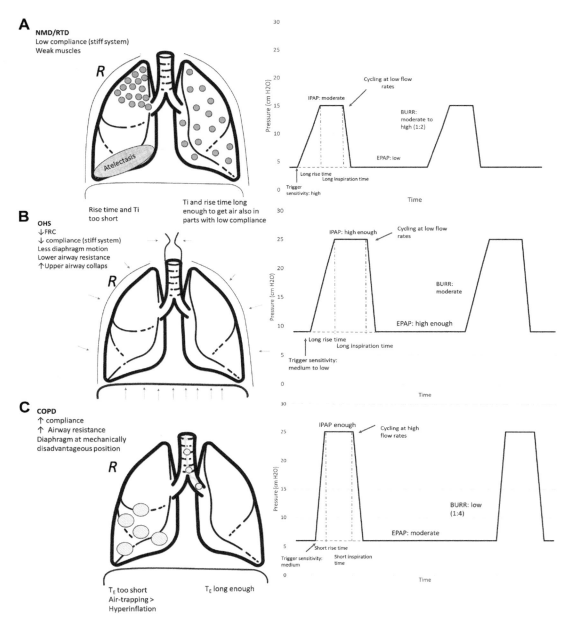

Fig. 1. Illustration of the consequences of incorrect (right lung, R) and correct (left lung, L) NIV settings in NMD (*A*), OHS (*B*) and COPD (*C*). For NMD (*top panel*) and COPD (*lowest panel*), it is shown what happens with inhaled air (NMD, blue circles) and exhaled air (COPD, yellow striped circles) if settings are not correct (*right lung, R*) and what if this is corrected (*left lung*). BURR, back-up respiratory rate; COPD, chronic obstructive pulmonary disease; EPAP, expiratory positive airway pressure; FRC, functional residual capacity; IPAP, inspiratory positive airway pressure; NMD, neuromuscular disease; OHS, obesity hypoventilation syndrome; RTD, restrictive thoracic disease; TE, expiratory time; Ti, inspiratory time.

such as MND/amyotrophic lateral sclerosis (ALS), it is recommended that NIV be started prior to the development of symptoms of hypoventilation, as this may lead to a slower decline of respiratory muscle strength and may also improve survival.[16] To detect deterioration early in these patients, a French expert panel proposed a 3 monthly assessment of symptoms of dyspnea and orthopnea, lung function (forced vital capacity in both sitting and lying positions), and respiratory muscle function (maximal inspiratory pressure [PImax], sniff nasal inspiratory pressure, and peak cough flow). Assessing gas exchange via arterial or capillary gas measurement was also recommended if the vital capacity is below 80% of predicted; if the PImax is below 60% predicted; if venous bicarbonate is above 28 mmol/L; if vital capacity measurements are unreliable; or on the basis of clinical signs or symptoms of concern.[17] In contrast to older guidelines emphasizing objective criteria such as pulmonary function tests and awake gas exchange parameters,[18,19] the French proposal places a greater emphasis on starting NIV based on symptoms, with objective assessment used only when clinical parameters such as orthopnea and severe dyspnea are absent.[17] Similarly, a recent Swiss guideline advocated early commencement of NIV, warning against waiting for daytime hypercapnia to develop, and suggesting signs and symptoms of orthopnea and dyspnea as being the most important criteria on which to base decisions around starting NIV.[17,20] Moreover, if objective criteria are needed, nocturnal monitoring should carry more weight than awake gas exchange as a substantial proportion of patients with NMD and normal awake blood gases will hypoventilate during sleep. Early monitoring of nocturnal transcutaneous CO_2 (PtCO_2) identifies patients with NMD at risk for needing home mechanical ventilation in the following 2 or more years.[21]

How to Start Non-invasive Ventilation in Neuromuscular Disease?

When starting NIV in NMD, it must be remembered that the primary pathology is respiratory muscle weakness, with accompanying thoracic deformities creating decreased chest wall compliance. Respiratory muscle weakness predisposes patients to making ineffective respiratory efforts, so the trigger sensitivity on the NIV device needs to be high. Furthermore, to ensure adequate ventilation, setting a back-up respiratory rate is also advisable.[22] A spontaneous-timed mode (ST-mode) is therefore the setting of first choice. A recent study has shown that a preset target volume mode (in this case, intelligent volume-assured pressure support [iVAPS] mode) required a longer adaptation period compared to ST-mode and resulted in greater upper-airway instability in patients with bulbar ALS,[23] and therefore is not recommended in this population. However, there might be certain populations of patients with NMD, as well as some pediatric populations, with increased upper airway resistance, reduced respiratory muscle strength, and/or pulmonary restriction (eg, from scoliosis and obesity), that might benefit from a ventilation mode that provides a guaranteed volume and/or is able to auto-titrate expiratory positive airway pressure (EPAP). Individual consideration is needed.[24]

Low chest wall compliance often requires a longer inspiratory time (Ti) and a slow rise time, to ensure maximal tidal volume and to allow sufficient time to distribute ventilation in the lungs from the apex to the bases (see **Fig. 1**). Consequently, cycle sensitivity should be set low, so that inspiratory time is sufficiently long.

In addition to nocturnal NIV, mouth-piece ventilation can be considered for daytime use, if the patient becomes more ventilator dependent. This allows some rest time from the mask, while relieving daytime respiratory muscle work and dyspnea. This type of ventilation can also be used to perform airstacking.[25]

INITIATION OF NON-INVASIVE VENTILATION IN OBESITY HYPOVENTILATION SYNDROME

The pathophysiology of OHS, as described by Masa, incorporates 3 major mechanisms: (1) obesity-related changes in the respiratory system; (2) alterations in respiratory drive; and (3) breathing abnormalities during sleep.[26] Excess abdominal and thoracic adipose tissue reduces functional residual capacity, impedes diaphragmatic motion, reduces compliance of the respiratory system, and augments lower airway resistance. Premature closing of small airways induces intrinsic positive end-expiratory pressure (PEEPi) and favors ventilation-perfusion (V/Q) mismatching. These detrimental mechanics should be counterbalanced by an increased respiratory drive. However, in patients with OHS, central hypoventilation and secondary depression of respiratory centers occurs.[27] Finally, 90% of patients with OHS have obstructive sleep apnea (OSA) due to excessive fat deposition around the upper airway, reduced lung volume, and fluid overload.[26] Patients with OHS and concomitant severe OSA should initially be treated with continuous positive airway pressure (CPAP), with evidence showing this to be noninferior to NIV in this population.[28,29] Patients without concomitant severe OSA should be offered NIV.[30]

Timing of Non-invasive Ventilation

Unfortunately, NIV is frequently initiated in OHS after an acute decompensation event with respiratory failure and right heart decompensation precipitates a hospital admission. In this situation, acute NIV is often needed to stabilize the patient. Moreover, discharging these patients with long-term NIV seems to be beneficial, as this strategy reduces mortality.[31] Once the patients are stabilized and their CO_2 has normalized, those patients identified as having the severe OSA/OHS phenotype may be able to be switched to CPAP.[32]

Starting NIV electively in a "stable" patient has clear advantages. First, presenting earlier avoids the risks (and costs) associated with acute decompensation. Second, there is an opportunity to discuss NIV treatment in the context of being part of a multidisciplinary treatment path with therapy options directed toward a healthy lifestyle, including weight loss, thus allowing engagement of the individual patient in their own care. In ambulatory OHS patients, achieving sufficient weight loss to reverse hypoventilation is difficult with lifestyle interventions alone[33]; so NIV will be advised anyway. In addition, when NIV is started in minimally symptomatic stable patients, adherence to therapy is low.[34] Therefore, we recommend commencing long-term NIV in patients with OHS with clear symptoms of nocturnal hypoventilation and integrating this process into a multidisciplinary clinic setting that includes a concomitant rehabilitation program directed toward a sustainable change in lifestyle,[35] regardless of whether the patient presents with acute or chronic respiratory failure.

How to Start Non-invasive Ventilation in Obesity Hypoventilation Syndrome?

In patients with OHS, pulmonary mechanics change during sleep depending on body position and sleep stage. To counterbalance the resulting fluctuations in delivered tidal volume, manufacturers have developed modes of ventilation that target delivery of a preset volume by automatically adjusting pressure support. It is also possible to set many NIV devices to auto-titrate EPAP so as to maintain a patent upper airway at comfortable pressures. Although conceptually interesting, studies have shown that gas exchange, sleep quality, and health-related quality of life improve similarly, regardless of whether an ST-mode with fixed pressures or an auto-titrating mode employing a preset target volume (average-volume-assured pressure support [AVAPS] or iVAPS mode) with or without auto-titration of EPAP (AVAPS-AE) is used.[36–40]

Patients with OHS often need high pressures to both maintain upper airway patency (sufficient EPAP) and to adequately ventilate a system with reduced compliance. A sufficiently high back-up respiratory rate is also necessary to ensure minute ventilation is maintained during periods of central hypoventilation.[41] One study found that patients who relied on a higher percentage of machine-triggered breaths during sleep had better outcomes.[36] Setting a longer Ti along with a slower rise time is also recommended to allow sufficient time to ventilate a system with low compliance.

INITIATION OF NON-INVASIVE VENTILATION IN CHRONIC OBSTRUCTIVE PULMONARY DISEASE

The cohort of patients with COPD who develop chronic hypercapnic respiratory failure encompasses a wide variety of COPD phenotypes, ranging from very severe COPD (with forced expiratory lung volumes of usually < 800 mL) to patients with overlap syndromes with concomitant obesity and/or OSA. It is important to recognize these different phenotypes, as the pathophysiology explaining respiratory failure may differ, impacting on the way therapy is applied. Furthermore, the phenotype seems to affect outcome.[42]

The use of NIV in COPD has long been controversial. However, more contemporary studies titrating NIV to optimize CO_2 have demonstrated clear benefits with respect to improvements in gas exchange, health-related quality of life and survival.[6,7] Consequently, NIV in patients with COPD with stable or persistent hypercapnic respiratory failure has now been incorporated into a number of clinical practice guidelines.[43,44] The beneficial effect from NIV reported by patients with COPD is partly explained by the improvement in symptoms related to nocturnal hypoventilation, such as non-restorative sleep, fatigue, and poor mental performance.[45] It should be noted that the effect of nocturnal NIV on symptoms of daytime dyspnea during unassisted breathing is minimal.[46]

Before Commencing Non-invasive Ventilation

The decision to start chronic NIV in COPD should be, as in any other disease, taken after carefully considering objective criteria (persistent or chronic hypercapnia, ie, $Paco_2 > 45$ mm Hg), the patient's own expectations and motivation, their social circumstances, and other potential treatment options. A systematic approach to consider the individual's COPD phenotype and so called "treatable traits" is also advised to determine what other treatment options should be added.[47] Combining the initiation of home NIV with a multidisciplinary pulmonary rehabilitation program augments outcomes and ensures that rehabilitation benefits can be sustained longer.[45,48] Before commencing NIV, our practice is to phenotype patients carefully, thereby gaining insight into comorbidities and lung function parameters such as the degree of airflow obstruction and hyperinflation. Moreover, as NIV will be lifelong in most patients and prognosis is generally poor,[49] it is advisable to start advanced care planning discussions when long-term NIV is started and to continue these discussions over the course of patient care.[50] While advanced care planning in other diseases such as cancer and ALS is common, this is often under-valued and under-recognized in COPD.[51] However, in the context of high symptom burden and poor prognosis, it is well worthwhile in these patients.

How to Start Non-invasive Ventilation in Chronic Obstructive Pulmonary Disease?

When setting up NIV in patients with COPD, the following general considerations are important. First, sufficient pressure support is needed to improve ventilation, recognizing that a proportion of the tidal volume delivered will ventilate regions of the lungs with high dead space which contribute very little to effective ventilation. Therefore, monitoring of gas exchange is essential. Second, lung mechanics in patients with COPD are characterized by small airways obstruction, gas trapping and hyperinflation, necessitating a long expiratory time on the ventilator settings. This can be achieved by aiming for controlled ventilation with a low back up rate and by limiting Ti. In many patients, careful up-titration of inspiratory positive airway pressure (IPAP) will lead to a low respiratory frequency and an increased proportion of controlled breaths. To achieve a higher tidal volume with a short Ti, a short rise time is also recommended. Third, PEEPi increases the likelihood of ineffective inspiratory efforts, as the patient first needs to overcome PEEPi before they can trigger the ventilator. Therefore, to counterbalance PEEPi, careful titration of EPAP is necessary.

Because of the diversity of the population with COPD starting on NIV, individual titration of NIV settings, taking into consideration individual patient traits, is necessary. For example, a patient with COPD with severe emphysema, severe airflow obstruction, and severe hyperinflation will benefit from a ventilatory strategy with a sufficiently high IPAP, low BURR, short Ti, short rise time, and adequate EPAP to prevent ineffective efforts. In contrast, a patient with moderately severe COPD, mild-to-moderate hyperinflation, concomitant obesity, and sleep apnea, will probably benefit from settings with sufficiently high IPAP, a slightly higher BURR, a slightly longer Ti, and a moderate rise time, with adequate EPAP to counterbalance upper airway obstruction.

When the above-mentioned considerations are taken into account, suitable modes of ventilation are the ST mode or pressure-controlled mode (PC mode; which gives even greater opportunity to control Ti), as well as volume-targeted modes of ventilation. To date, no studies have shown a clear benefit of one mode over another in patient with COPD.[52–54]

MONITORING DURING THE INITIATION PHASE

A wide variety of clinical and ventilatory parameters are monitored during the initiation phase. However, recent studies have demonstrated comparable outcomes whether initiating NIV in the patient's home or during more intensive and complex in-hospital care.[55,56] These findings question the need to carry out extensive monitoring of different ventilator parameters during the initial acclimation period. This approach must be balanced against the need for careful titration of NIV, including physiologic parameters, and ensuring adequate training of the patient and carers in their understanding and skills in how to use the ventilator, in order to achieve successful and comfortable ventilation in the longer term.

Several objective physiologic data can be monitored. First, data collected from the ventilator itself, such as usage hours, leakage, tidal volumes, respiratory frequency, apnea/hypopnea indices, and Ti, can be retrieved. Many devices now also allow access to ventilator data via online platforms. Patient–ventilator asynchrony (PVA) can, in general, be detected from breath-by-breath flow and pressure curve data, although some asynchrony might be misclassified or missed.[57] Second, to ensure that optimization of alveolar ventilation is achieved, we recommend monitoring gas exchange, either by awake arterial or capillary blood gas analyses, or by nocturnal transcutaneous O_2 and CO_2 monitoring.[58] Patients with COPD can be well ventilated during sleep, but still present with hypercapnia during wakefulness due to their advanced lung disease. Third, polysomnographic (PSG) monitoring can be used to initiate NIV, allowing titration of settings to optimize the reduction in respiratory events, improve sleep quality,[59] and more precisely recognize and manage PVA.[57] It is worth noting that in patients with COPD/overlap syndrome, it has been shown that nurse-led titration of settings guided by ventilator data and nocturnal transcutaneous monitoring eventually results in similar or even better outcomes compared to more sophisticated PSG titration.[60] Finally, new tools are now available that might simplify monitoring further, for example, wearables. The value of these devices need to be established in patients with chronic respiratory failure. In **Fig. 2**, an algorithm is proposed for monitoring during the initiation phase.

Where to Initiate Non-invasive Ventilation?

NIV can be initiated in any location where a comfortable, safe environment can be assured. Whether this is in the hospital, the outpatient clinic,

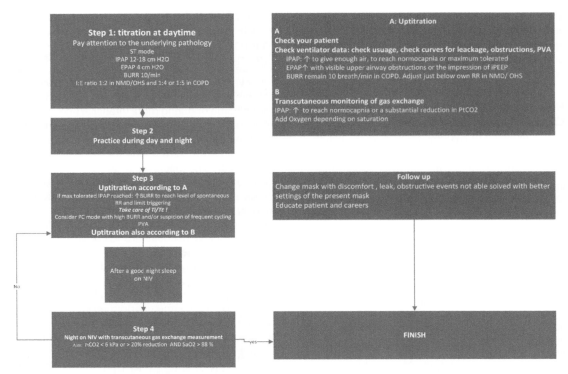

Fig. 2. Practical guide to initiating long-term NIV. BURR, back-up respiratory rate; COPD, chronic obstructive pulmonary disease; EPAP, expiratory positive airway pressure; IPAP, inspiratory positive airway pressure; NMD, neuromuscular disease; OHS, obesity hypoventilation syndrome; PEEPi, intrinsic PEEP; PtCO$_2$, transcutaneously measured partial carbon dioxide (CO$_2$) pressure; PVA, patient-ventilator asynchrony; RR, respiratory rate; SaO$_2$, oxygen saturation; ST-mode, spontaneous-timed mode.

or at home is probably not the main factor determining NIV success. Careful titration of ventilator settings, optimal mask fitting, and education of the patient and family are the cornerstones of successful continuation of NIV treatment.

The last decade has seen a transition from in-hospital to outpatient and at-home initiation of NIV. Health care resources for elective admission of stable patients for commencement of NIV is limited in most countries, while many patients consider in-hospital initiation of NIV to be stressful. Patients prefer to commence NIV in their own environment, where they have their own care team and can acclimatize to therapy at their own pace.[61] Furthermore, limited hospital bed capacity for elective admissions can delay the initiation of NIV, putting more severe patients at an increased risk of acute decompensation and mortality.[55] By initiating NIV at-home, intervention can occur earlier, which is especially preferable for patients with more rapidly progressive disorders.

Several recent studies have shown that initiating long-term NIV at home using telemonitoring of ventilator data, measurement of transcutaneous gas exchange parameters, and daily nurse-led

adjustments of the ventilator settings to be noninferior to in-hospital NIV initiation in patients with chronic respiratory failure, irrespective of the primary disease process.[56,62,63] Furthermore, compared to several days of in-hospital initiation, direct costs of this approach are considerably lower. However, this approach requires an organizational structure where clinicians initiating NIV can visit the patient at home as needed, for as long as needed, using a reliable and preferably integrated telemonitoring system. While there is some debate around the necessity for home gas exchange assessment, this likely depends on the patient's underlying disease. In a retrospective trial of patients with ALS, use of telemonitored ventilator data only to initiate NIV in the patient's home produced favorable outcomes, with significantly more patients adherent to NIV at 30 days compared to in-hospital initiation.[64] Nevertheless, it must be borne in mind that with home initiation of NIV, more burden of care in the early phase of therapy is shifted to the caregivers, as they learn how to manage the mask and ventilator, and how to troubleshoot problems arising from the application of therapy. This highlights the need for a comprehensive training program with sufficient time and resources allocated to its delivery.

An alternative system enabling home initiation of NIV might be the use of automatic titrating systems, such as volume-assured auto-EPAP titrating modes. A recent randomized study found similar clinical effectiveness using auto-titrating NIV at home, combined with oximetry, compared to in-hospital overnight attended titration of fixed pressure NIV in stable OHS patients.[64] However, those allocated to home setup with an autotitrating NIV device required more non-planned visits, more phone calls, and more frequent ventilator setting changes due to technical and medical problems compared to outpatient initiation with auto-titration of pressures.[65] It should be noted, however, that a remote monitoring system capable of recording data and changing device settings via an on-line platform was not used in this study. The use of this technology in conjunction with autotitration of device settings may have simplified the acclimation process and reduced the need for more health care contact. In considering home auto-titration of NIV settings, attention to mask fit, monitoring of therapy effectiveness, and education of the patient and family remain the most important components of successful therapy initiation.

In situations where home initiation of NIV may not be feasible, outpatient daytime set-up is an option.[55,66,67] However, repeated training and monitoring sessions supervised by a professional may be required,[68] and it may not be possible to capture a period of sleep during the daytime titration process. Returning to an outpatient clinic over several sessions to initiate NIV can be a significant burden for severely disabled patients and their families. Therefore, a more flexible approach to care is need, for example, combining a single outpatient acclimatization and mask fitting session with several days of nocturnal home telemonitoring in conjunction with video consultations, might combine efficiency (especially for health care providers) with efficacy and ease (for patients).

SUMMARY

Initiation of long-term NIV requires careful consideration of the patient's condition, taking into account the underlying disease causing chronic respiratory failure, as well as the patient's and caregivers' motivation and expectations, wishes and social circumstances. The decision to eventually start NIV hinges on a combination of objective signs and symptoms of nocturnal hypoventilation, in the context of the trajectory and prognosis of the underlying disease. A good understanding of

the underlying pathophysiology leads to a systematic and balanced approach to NIV titration. Ultimately, the location where NIV is initiated is not as critical as that location being a comfortable, safe environment where adequate monitoring can be provided. With this in mind, home initiation of long-term NIV has many advantages and is the preferred approach to begin treatment for the majority of patients with chronic respiratory failure.

CLINICS CARE POINTS

- Inform patients and relatives well about expected benefits and potential drawbacks of intiating chronic home NIV.

- If possible, give patients and relatives time to consider their decision to start chronic NIV carefully.

- Base the decision to start chronic NIV on a combination of objective signs of hypoventilation and subjective symptoms, taking into account the underlying disease and evidence base in this disease group.

- In patients with neuromuscular diseases, chronic NIV settings should be titrated counterbalancing the primary pathophysiology, ie, respiratory muscle weakness with a decreased chest wall compliance, with high trigger sensitivity, a back-up respiratory rate, a longer inspiratory time, a slow rise time, and low cycle sensitivity.

- In patients with OHS, sufficient expiratory pressure is needed to maintain upper airway patency, and sufficient inspiratory pressure is needed to ventilate a system with low chest wall compliance.

- In OHS, Auto-titrating modes might help to adjust in- and expiratory pressure depending on changing pulmonary mechanics depending on body position and sleep stage.

- In patients with COPD, as dead space ventilation is high, sufficient inspiratory pressure is needed to achieve effective correction of alveolar ventilation.

- In COPD, a low back-up respiratory rate is advised, with a short inspiratory time and fast rise time, so that suffient expiratory time assures optimal lung emptying during expiration.

- Start chronic NIV always in a safe and comfortable environment where appropriate monitoring is available.

- Monitor patients being on NIV to ensure effective and comfortable ventilation.

DISCLOSURE

During the preparation of this work the authors did not use any AI and AI-assisted technologies in the writing process, except from endnote to order the references.

REFERENCES

1. Simonds AK. Recent advances in respiratory care for neuromuscular disease. Chest 2006;130(6):1879–86.
2. Bourke SC, Bullock RE, Williams TL, et al. Noninvasive ventilation in ALS: indications and effect on quality of life. Neurology 2003;61(2):171–7.
3. Annane D, Orlikowski D, Chevret S. Nocturnal mechanical ventilation for chronic hypoventilation in patients with neuromuscular and chest wall disorders. Cochrane Database Syst Rev 2014;2014(12): Cd001941.
4. Bourke SC, Tomlinson M, Williams TL, et al. Effects of non-invasive ventilation on survival and quality of life in patients with amyotrophic lateral sclerosis: a randomised controlled trial. Lancet Neurol 2006;5(2): 140–7.
5. Afshar M, Brozek JL, Soghier I, et al. The role of positive airway pressure therapy in adults with obesity hypoventilation syndrome. a systematic review and meta-analysis. Ann Am Thorac Soc 2020;17(3):344–60.
6. Köhnlein T, Windisch W, Köhler D, et al. Non-invasive positive pressure ventilation for the treatment of severe stable chronic obstructive pulmonary disease: a prospective, multicentre, randomised, controlled clinical trial. Lancet Respir Med 2014;2(9):698–705.
7. Murphy PB, Rehal S, Arbane G, et al. Effect of home noninvasive ventilation with oxygen therapy vs oxygen therapy alone on hospital readmission or death after an acute COPD exacerbation: a randomized clinical trial. JAMA 2017;317(21):2177–86.
8. Chatwin M, Simonds AK. Long-term mechanical insufflation-exsufflation cough assistance in neuromuscular disease: patterns of use and lessons for application. Respir Care 2020;65(2):135–43.
9. Bento J, Gonçalves M, Silva N, et al. Indications and compliance of home mechanical insufflation-exsufflation in patients with neuromuscular diseases. Arch Bronconeumol 2010;46(8):420–5.
10. Toussaint M, Chatwin M, Soudon P. Mechanical ventilation in Duchenne patients with chronic respiratory insufficiency: clinical implications of 20 years published experience. Chron Respir Dis 2007;4(3): 167–77.
11. Barry C, Larner E, Copsey H, et al. Non-invasive ventilation support for people with amyotrophic lateral sclerosis: multidisciplinary team management. Curr Opin Support Palliat Care 2021;15(4):214–8.
12. Baxter SK, Johnson M, Clowes M, et al. Optimizing the noninvasive ventilation pathway for patients with amyotrophic lateral sclerosis/motor neuron disease: a systematic review. Amyotroph Lateral Scler Frontotemporal Degener 2019;20(7–8):461–72.
13. Mercadante S, Al-Husinat L. Palliative care in amyotrophic lateral sclerosis. J Pain Symptom Manage 2023;66(4):e485–99.
14. Seijger C, Raaphorst J, Vonk J, et al. New Insights in Adherence and Survival in Myotonic Dystrophy Patients Using Home Mechanical Ventilation. Respiration 2021;100(2):154–63.
15. Vosse BAH, Seijger C, Cobben N, et al. Noninvasive Home Mechanical Ventilation in Adult Myotonic Dystrophy Type 1: A Systematic Review. Respiration 2021;100(8):816–25.
16. Sarasate M, González N, Córdoba-Izquierdo A, et al. Impact of early non-invasive ventilation in amyotrophic lateral sclerosis: a multicenter randomized controlled trial. J Neuromuscul Dis 2023;10(4): 627–37.
17. Georges M, Perez T, Rabec C, et al. Proposals from a French expert panel for respiratory care in ALS patients. Respir Med Res 2022;81:100901.
18. Andersen PM, Abrahams S, Borasio GD, et al. EFNS guidelines on the clinical management of amyotrophic lateral sclerosis (MALS)–revised report of an EFNS task force. Eur J Neurol 2012;19(3):360–75.
19. Miller RG, Brooks BR, Swain-Eng RJ, et al. Quality improvement in neurology: amyotrophic lateral sclerosis quality measures: report of the quality measurement and reporting subcommittee of the American Academy of Neurology. Neurology 2013; 81(24):2136–40.
20. Janssens JP, Michel F, Schwarz EI, et al. Long-term mechanical ventilation: recommendations of the swiss society of pulmonology. Respiration 2020;1–36.
21. Orlikowski D, Prigent H, Quera Salva MA, et al. Prognostic value of nocturnal hypoventilation in neuromuscular patients. Neuromuscul Disord 2017; 27(4):326–30.
22. Vrijsen B, Buyse B, Belge C, et al. Randomized cross-over trial of ventilator modes during noninvasive ventilation titration in amyotrophic lateral sclerosis. Respirology 2017;22(6):1212–8.
23. Panyarath P, Adam V, Kimoff RJ, et al. Alveolar ventilation-targeted versus spontaneous/timed mode for home noninvasive ventilation in amyotrophic lateral sclerosis. Respir Care 2022;67(9):1109–20.
24. Cithiravel N, Xiao L, Shi J, et al. Volume assured pressure support mode use for non-invasive ventilation in pediatrics. Pediatr Pulmonol 2023;59(1):7–18.
25. Toussaint M, Chatwin M, Gonçalves MR, et al. Mouthpiece ventilation in neuromuscular disorders: narrative review of technical issues important for clinical success. Respir Med 2021;180:106373.
26. Masa JF, Pépin JL, Borel JC, et al. Obesity hypoventilation syndrome. Eur Respir Rev 2019;28(151): 180097.

27. Piper AJ, Grunstein RR. Big breathing: the complex interaction of obesity, hypoventilation, weight loss, and respiratory function. J Appl Physiol (1985) 2010;108(1):199–205.

28. Masa JF, Corral J, Alonso ML, et al. Efficacy of different treatment alternatives for obesity hypoventilation syndrome. pickwick study. Am J Respir Crit Care Med 2015;192(1):86–95.

29. López-Jiménez MJ, Masa JF, Corral J, et al. Mid- and long-term efficacy of non-invasive ventilation in obesity hypoventilation syndrome: the pickwick's study. Arch Bronconeumol 2016;52(3):158–65.

30. Masa JF, Corral J, Caballero C, et al. Non-invasive ventilation in obesity hypoventilation syndrome without severe obstructive sleep apnoea. Thorax 2016;71(10):899–906.

31. Mokhlesi B, Masa JF, Afshar M, et al. The effect of hospital discharge with empiric noninvasive ventilation on mortality in hospitalized patients with obesity hypoventilation syndrome. an individual patient data meta-analysis. Ann Am Thorac Soc 2020;17(5):627–37.

32. Arellano-Maric MP, Hamm C, Duiverman ML, et al. Obesity hypoventilation syndrome treated with non-invasive ventilation: is a switch to CPAP therapy feasible? Respirology 2020;25(4):435–42.

33. Kakazu MT, Soghier I, Afshar M, et al. Weight loss interventions as treatment of obesity hypoventilation syndrome. a systematic review. Ann Am Thorac Soc 2020;17(4):492–502.

34. Cheng MCF, Murphy PB, Lee K, et al. Screening and treatment of pre-bariatric surgical patients with obesity related sleep disordered breathing. J Thorac Dis 2023;15(7):4066–73.

35. Mandal S, Suh ES, Harding R, et al. Nutrition and exercise rehabilitation in obesity hypoventilation syndrome (NERO): a pilot randomised controlled trial. Thorax 2018;73(1):62–9.

36. Murphy PB, Davidson C, Hind MD, et al. Volume targeted versus pressure support non-invasive ventilation in patients with super obesity and chronic respiratory failure: a randomised controlled trial. Thorax 2012;67(8):727–34.

37. Patout M, Gagnadoux F, Rabec C, et al. AVAPS-AE versus ST mode: a randomized controlled trial in patients with obesity hypoventilation syndrome. Respirology 2020;25(10):1073–81.

38. Storre JH, Seuthe B, Fiechter R, et al. Average volume-assured pressure support in obesity hypoventilation: a randomized crossover trial. Chest 2006;130(3):815–21.

39. Janssens JP, Metzger M, Sforza E. Impact of volume targeting on efficacy of bi-level non-invasive ventilation and sleep in obesity-hypoventilation. Respir Med 2009;103(2):165–72.

40. Xu J, Wei Z, Li W, et al. Effect of different modes of positive airway pressure treatment on obesity hypoventilation syndrome: a systematic review and network meta-analysis. Sleep Med 2022;91:51–8.

41. Contal O, Adler D, Borel JC, et al. Impact of different backup respiratory rates on the efficacy of noninvasive positive pressure ventilation in obesity hypoventilation syndrome: a randomized trial. Chest 2013;143(1):37–46.

42. Janssens JP, Cantero C, Pasquina P, et al. Long-term noninvasive ventilation in chronic obstructive pulmonary disease: association between clinical phenotypes and survival. Respiration 2022;101(10):939–47.

43. Ergan B, Oczkowski S, Rochwerg B, et al. European Respiratory Society guidelines on long-term home non-invasive ventilation for management of COPD. Eur Respir J 2019;54(3):1901003.

44. Macrea M, Oczkowski S, Rochwerg B, et al. Long-term noninvasive ventilation in chronic stable hypercapnic chronic obstructive pulmonary disease. an official american thoracic society clinical practice guideline. Am J Respir Crit Care Med 2020;202(4):e74–87.

45. Duiverman ML, Wempe JB, Bladder G, et al. Nocturnal non-invasive ventilation in addition to rehabilitation in hypercapnic patients with COPD. Thorax 2008;63(12):1052–7.

46. Raveling T, Vonk J, Struik FM, et al. Chronic non-invasive ventilation for chronic obstructive pulmonary disease. Cochrane Database Syst Rev 2021;8(8):Cd002878.

47. van Dijk M, Gan CT, Koster TD, et al. Treatment of severe stable COPD: the multidimensional approach of treatable traits. ERJ Open Res 2020;6(3):00322–2019.

48. Duiverman ML, Wempe JB, Bladder G, et al. Two-year home-based nocturnal noninvasive ventilation added to rehabilitation in chronic obstructive pulmonary disease patients: a randomized controlled trial. Respir Res 2011;12(1):112.

49. Patout M, Lhuillier E, Kaltsakas G, et al. Long-term survival following initiation of home non-invasive ventilation: a European study. Thorax 2020;75(11):965–73.

50. Raveling T, Rantala HA, Duiverman ML. Home ventilation for patients with end-stage chronic obstructive pulmonary disease. Curr Opin Support Palliat Care 2023;17(4):277–82.

51. Janssen DJA, Bajwah S, Boon MH, et al. European Respiratory Society clinical practice guideline: palliative care for people with COPD or interstitial lung disease. Eur Respir J 2023;62(2):2202014.

52. Ekkernkamp E, Storre JH, Windisch W, et al. Impact of intelligent volume-assured pressure support on sleep quality in stable hypercapnic chronic obstructive pulmonary disease patients: a randomized, crossover study. Respiration 2014;88(4):270–6.

53. Storre JH, Matrosovich E, Ekkernkamp E, et al. Home mechanical ventilation for COPD: high-intensity versus target volume noninvasive ventilation. Respir Care 2014;59(9):1389–97.

54. Oscroft NS, Chadwick R, Davies MG, et al. Volume assured versus pressure preset non-invasive ventilation for compensated ventilatory failure in COPD. Respir Med 2014;108(10):1508–15.

55. Sheers N, Berlowitz DJ, Rautela L, et al. Improved survival with an ambulatory model of non-invasive ventilation implementation in motor neuron disease. Amyotroph Lateral Scler Frontotemporal Degener 2014;15(3–4):180–4.

56. Duiverman ML, Vonk JM, Bladder G, et al. Home initiation of chronic non-invasive ventilation in COPD patients with chronic hypercapnic respiratory failure: a randomised controlled trial. Thorax 2020;75(3):244–52.

57. Gonzalez-Bermejo J, Janssens JP, Rabec C, et al. Framework for patient-ventilator asynchrony during long-term non-invasive ventilation. Thorax 2019;74(7):715–7.

58. Hazenberg A, Zijlstra JG, Kerstjens HA, et al. Validation of a transcutaneous CO(2) monitor in adult patients with chronic respiratory failure. Respiration 2011;81(3):242–6.

59. Vrijsen B, Testelmans D, Belge C, et al. Patient-ventilator asynchrony, leaks and sleep in patients with amyotrophic lateral sclerosis. Amyotroph Lateral Scler Frontotemporal Degener 2016;17(5–6):343–50.

60. Patout M, Arbane G, Cuvelier A, et al. Polysomnography versus limited respiratory monitoring and nurse-led titration to optimise non-invasive ventilation set-up: a pilot randomised clinical trial. Thorax 2019;74(1):83–6.

61. Ribeiro C, Jácome C, Oliveira P, et al. Patients experience regarding home mechanical ventilation in an outpatient setting. Chron Respir Dis 2022;19. 14799731221137082.

62. van den Biggelaar RJM, Hazenberg A, Cobben NAM, et al. A Randomized Trial of Initiation of Chronic Noninvasive Mechanical Ventilation at Home vs In-Hospital in Patients With Neuromuscular Disease and Thoracic Cage Disorder: The Dutch Homerun Trial. Chest 2020;158(6):2493–501.

63. Hazenberg A, Kerstjens HA, Prins SC, et al. Initiation of home mechanical ventilation at home: a randomised controlled trial of efficacy, feasibility and costs. Respir Med 2014;108(9):1387–95.

64. Réginault T, Bouteleux B, Wibart P, et al. At-home noninvasive ventilation initiation with telemonitoring in amyotrophic lateral sclerosis patients: a retrospective study. ERJ Open Res 2023;9(1):00438–2022.

65. Murphy PB, Patout M, Arbane G, et al. Cost-effectiveness of outpatient versus inpatient non-invasive ventilation setup in obesity hypoventilation syndrome: the OPIP trial. Thorax 2023;78(1):24–31.

66. Sheers N, Howard ME, Berlowitz DJ. Ambulatory adaptation of non-invasive ventilation in motor neuron disease: where limits of effectiveness end–reply. Amyotroph Lateral Scler Frontotemporal Degener 2015;16(1–2):139–40.

67. Chatwin M, Nickol AH, Morrell MJ, et al. Randomised trial of inpatient versus outpatient initiation of home mechanical ventilation in patients with nocturnal hypoventilation. Respir Med 2008;102(11):1528–35.

68. Volpato E, Vitacca M, Ptacinsky L, et al. Home-based adaptation to night-time non-invasive ventilation in patients with amyotrophic lateral sclerosis: a randomized controlled trial. J Clin Med 2022;11(11):3178.

Interfaces for Home Noninvasive Ventilation

Amanda J. Piper, BAppSc, MEd, PhD

KEYWORDS

- Hypercapnia • Masks • Noninvasive ventilation • Leak • Sleep hypoventilation

KEY POINTS

- Interface choice is a critical consideration for home noninvasive ventilation (NIV).
- Both patient-related and equipment-related factors need to be considered when choosing a style of interface for NIV.
- Oronasal masks are now the most common interface used during sleep.
- While randomized trials have failed to find major differences in clinical outcomes between nasal and oronasal masks, significant differences in individual responses to these masks occur.

INTRODUCTION

Noninvasive ventilation (NIV) has been a major advance in the management of people with respiratory insufficiency. The interface used for NIV forms a vital link between the ventilator device and the respiratory system of the individual, and figures prominently in the success and safety of establishing therapy, especially in the setting of long-term home ventilation. This article reviews the types of interfaces used for long-term NIV, factors influencing the choice of an interface for a particular individual, and some of the more common issues and side effects related to interface use.

CHOOSING AN APPROPRIATE MASK: CLINICAL CONSIDERATIONS

A personalized approach to mask selection is required, considering a range of patient-related and equipment-related issues to maximize comfort and acceptance of therapy (**Box 1**). For most home NIV users, a nasal or oronasal mask will be prescribed, at least when therapy is used primarily during sleep.[1–3] Both nasal and oronasal masks place some pressure over the nasal bridge, which is a common point for skin and tissue damage,

especially with prolonged use. More recently, hybrid oronasal masks have been introduced. These masks cover the mouth, but the top edge of the interface sits along the bottom of the nose, thereby avoiding contact with the nasal bridge. Full face masks, which enclose the entire front of the face including the eyes, are an option for home ventilation for both nocturnal and daytime use[1,4] (**Fig. 1**). At the other extreme are the nasal pillows or cushions that cover the nostrils or bottom of the nose only, leaving both the nasal bridge and mouth free. Oral interfaces are also available, with mouthpiece ventilation a common option for daytime ventilatory support.[1,5]

Home NIV masks can either to be vented, incorporating a calibrated intentional leak built into the mask frame for clearance of carbon dioxide, or non-vented, where an active expiratory valve or separate expiratory respiratory limb directs exhaled gas out of the respiratory circuit. Vented masks with a single limb circuit are now the most common set up for home NIV.[1,2]

The range of commercially available masks are generally sufficient to find an acceptable interface for most elderly patients. However, mask choices for infants and young children are more limited. Some time ago, customized masks were proposed to minimize leak and maximize fit and comfort.[6]

Department of Respiratory and Sleep Medicine, Respiratory Support Service, Level 11, E Block, Royal Prince Alfred Hospital, Missenden Road, Camperdown, New South Wales 2050, Australia
E-mail address: amanda.piper@health.nsw.gov.au

Sleep Med Clin 19 (2024) 431–441
https://doi.org/10.1016/j.jsmc.2024.04.005
1556-407X/24/© 2024 Elsevier Inc. All rights reserved.

<table>
<tr><td>

Box 1
Considerations when choosing an interface for home noninvasive ventilation

- Patient preference and comfort
- Facial anatomy
  - Available in a range of sizes to suit both narrow, elongated features as well as rounder, flatter features
  - Symmetry of features
  - Does not occlude nostrils
  - Minimizes pressure on soft tissue or bony structures such as the nasal bridge or dentition
- Preferred breathing route
  - Nasal patency
  - Ability to maintain lip closure
- Minimization of unintentional leak
- Mode of ventilation and respiratory circuit used
  - Vented or non-vented mask required
  - Satisfactory CO_2 clearance
- Ease of patient/carer placing and removing mask
- Pressures used during NIV
- Are extended periods of ventilation likely?
- Ability to maintain mask seal without over-tightening of headstraps
- Patient not allergic to the mask materials
- Stability of the interface with patient movement
- Clinician experience and skill in fitting the interface

</td></tr>
</table>

20 years a shift in prescribing practices has occurred. A recent international survey of long-term home NIV in restrictive thoracic disorders found oronasal and full-face masks were the preferred interface in this setting, with only 20% of patients using nasal masks or nasal pillows for sleep.[1] Similarly, a cross-sectional study of people with chronic obstructive pulmonary disease (COPD) found almost 80% used an oronasal mask.[3] This shift toward oronasal masks could reflect improvements in the design and range of oronasal masks now available or may simply reflect greater awareness of the impact unintentional leaks have on the efficacy of ventilation and sleep quality.[12,13] It has also been suggested that the increasing use of higher levels of inspiratory positive airway pressure (IPAP) to maximally reduce daytime CO_2 in patients with COPD[14–16] may have played a role.[3]

For patients requiring extended periods of ventilatory support, mouthpiece ventilation is a common approach,[1,17] where an angled mouthpiece or a "straw" connected to the distal end of the respiratory circuit is used to deliver ventilation (**Fig. 2**). This enables the individual to access ventilation on an "as needed" basis by placing their lips over or on the mouthpiece to trigger the device into inspiration.[17] However, patients with weak lip and neck muscles may not be able to grab and hold the mouthpiece.[17,18] For these individuals, other interfaces such as nasal pillows or hybrid oronasal masks may be used for daytime ventilation. Although uncommonly used now, mouthpiece ventilation, secured by a lip seal and strap, is also an option for sleep.[1] The key clinical point to highlight is the need to have alternative styles of masks available, especially when therapy is used on a more extended basis.

However, most home ventilation centers do not have access to the resources and skilled staff needed to produce customized masks for individual patients, and commercial masks have largely become the norm. With access to 3 dimensional scanning and printing now becoming more widely available, interest in customized masks and modifications has again increased.[7–9]

WHAT MASKS ARE CURRENTLY USED IN THE HOME SETTING?

A 2005 survey of long-term NIV practices found nasal masks were most often prescribed, irrespective of the patient's primary diagnosis,[10] with nasal masks considered better tolerated than oronasal masks or nasal pillows.[11] However, over the past

SECURING THE MASK—THE HEADGEAR

The headgear is designed to hold these masks in place (**Fig. 3**). Straps on the headgear are adjustable and usually come in several different sizes and configurations. When fitting and donning the headgear, care is needed to balance sufficient tightening of the straps to hold the mask securely in place without creating too much pressure on the face. Asymmetrical tension on the straps can leave the mask unevenly placed on the face, increasing the risk of leak and discomfort. Further, there is often a tendency pull the headstraps tighter to resolve leak, which simply deforms the mask cushion and increases the pressure exerted on the face. More appropriately, the mask should be repositioned or refitted. Like mask cushions, headstraps should be regularly cleaned and replaced to maintain best fit.

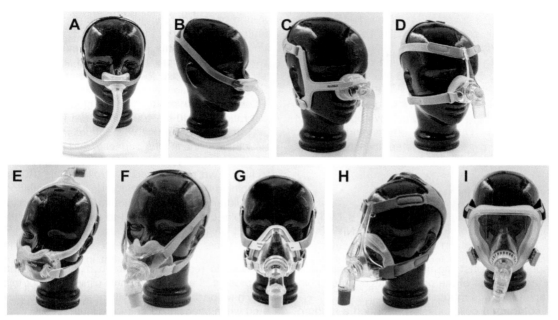

Fig. 1. Commercially available masks for long-term NIV are available in a range of styles including nasal pillows and prongs (*A, B*) nasal masks (*C, D*) hybrid masks which sit along the base of the nose and cover the mouth (*E, F*) oronasal masks (*G, H*) and total face masks (*I*). (*Courtesy of* Dr Collette Menadue and Dr Kerri Melehan)

For patients with limited upper limb function, the ease with which the mask can be sited and removed also needs to be considered. Magnetic clip attachments between the mask frame and headgear can be a useful option. However, there is a risk that the magnetic field associated with these magnets could cause problems with the operation of implantable medical devices such as pacemakers or movement of metallic objects like stents and clips, and therefore are contraindicated in these circumstances.

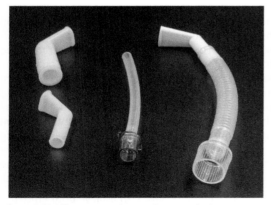

Fig. 2. Different styles of mouthpiece, most commonly used for daytime ventilatory support. (*Courtesy of* Dr Collette Menadue and Dr Kerri Melehan)

ARE THERE PHYSIOLOGIC OR CLINICAL DIFFERENCES BETWEEN NASAL AND ORONASAL MASKS?

Nasal masks are often perceived to be more comfortable[11,19,20] and may allow lower pressures for effective ventilation than oronasal masks,[19] the latter having been associated with upper airway obstruction.[21] However, unintentional leak from the mouth with nasal masks may reduce ventilation effectiveness and impair sleep quality.[12] Oronasal masks are more commonly used in patients with COPD when higher pressures are required[3] or when long-term NIV is commenced following an acute respiratory event.[22]

There have been limited studies comparing different mask types for home NIV (**Table 1**). Understanding potential differences in clinical response between mask styles is important when troubleshooting and considering switching masks for leak or discomfort. Willson and colleagues[20] randomized 16 participants with nocturnal hypoventilation established on long-term NIV to using either a nasal or oronasal mask during sleep over 2 consecutive nights in a sleep laboratory. While no difference in nocturnal gas exchange was seen, sleep efficiency was higher with nasal masks and there was a trend toward participants rating these as more comfortable. However, as participants were already established on nasal mask NIV, the single night protocol likely biased

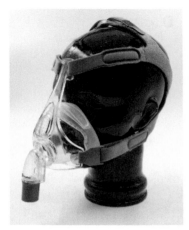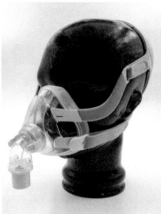

Fig. 3. Headstraps anchor the mask to the patient's face. Some configurations of headstrap may be more comfortable or stable for an individual. The straps can be held onto the mask frame with either plastic clips or magnetic studs, the latter often being easier to use for those with limited hand strength or dexterity. (*Courtesy of* Dr Collette Menadue and Dr Kerri Melehan)

responses against the unfamiliar oronasal mask. Furthermore, 14 of the participants required chinstraps to reduce mouth leak.

Leotard and colleagues[23] performed a randomized, crossover study of either 1 week use of nasal or oronasal masks in 30 home NIV-users with neuromuscular disorders. Overall, no significant difference in mean nocturnal oxyhemoglobin saturation (SpO_2) between interfaces was found. Both interfaces also performed similarly with respect to residual apnea hypopnea index, mean nocturnal transcutaneous CO_2 levels, time spent with SpO_2 less than 90%, time spent with leak and adherence to NIV. However, post hoc analysis showed a reduction in NIV efficacy and an increase in mask side effects during the transition to a new interface. Similarly, a randomized crossover trial in patients with COPD on home NIV showed both styles of mask successfully delivered therapy overnight with comparable mean levels of transcutaneous CO_2.[24] However, at an individual level, significant heterogeneity in sleep quality and gas exchange was observed. This highlights the need for closer monitoring of a patient upon switching mask styles.

In an individual participant data meta-analysis, Lebret and colleagues[25] compared nasal and oronasal masks on treatment efficacy and adherence in patients with COPD and obesity hypoventilation syndrome. The authors found no difference between mask types with respect to daytime arterial carbon dioxide ($Paco_2$), arterial oxygen (Pao_2), or NIV adherence, with no interaction between patient diagnosis and mask type for any outcome. However, while expiratory positive airway pressure levels were similar between masks, a higher mean IPAP was needed when using oronasal masks.

In summary, while no interface guarantees better ventilation or adherence to long-term NIV, significant within patient differences in comfort and

physiologic responses between mask styles can be present,[24] and the potential clinical impact this may have on the efficacy of NIV needs to be considered when choosing or changing interfaces.[23,26]

TECHNICAL CONSIDERATIONS WITH DIFFERENT INTERFACE TYPES
Effect of Leak on Ventilator Performance and Ventilation Efficacy

Most home NIV is delivered as pressure-targeted therapy using a single limb circuit with an expiratory vent integrated either into the circuit or, more commonly, within the interface itself[1] to minimize CO_2 rebreathing. The level of pressure set on the ventilator, the style of interface and the brand of the device will all influence the degree of intentional leak present,[27,28] with higher values expected with oronasal masks compared to nasal masks at the same pressure settings. Unintentional leaks are those that occur between the mask and skin or from the open mouth with nasal masks and pillows. Unintentional leaks may not be present when the patient is awake but can become substantial during sleep with loss of muscle tone.[29] Home ventilators are designed to compensate for some degree of unintentional leak by increasing the inspiratory flow to maintain set pressure. However, if these leaks are too high the comfort and effectiveness of NIV may be compromised (**Fig. 4**).

Ventilator performance can also be affected by large unintentional leaks, producing issues with inspiratory triggering and breath cycling, resulting in patient–ventilator asynchrony.[30,31] The magnitude of the leak, pattern of leakage[30] along with the mechanical properties of the lung and the patency of the upper airway all influence the likelihood of asynchrony occurring.[32] Sleep quality

Table 1
Studies comparing nasal and oronasal masks in chronic hypoventilation syndromes

Authors, Date	N	Study Population	Study Type	Outcomes Measures
Navalesi et al,[11] 2000	26	Stable hypercapnia, naïve to NIV	RXT, 30 min trials on each interface	Nasal mask better tolerated than ONM although $Paco_2$ was significantly higher (49.5±9.4 mm Hg vs 52.4 + 11 mm Hg) and tidal volume was lower.
Willson et al,[20] 2004	16	Established NIV-users	RXT, single night each arm	Reduced sleep efficiency with ONM. Similar AHI, TST minimum average SpO_2, delta NREM to REM $TcCO_2$. Chinstrap needed in 14 participants during NM use to minimize mouth leak
Fernandez et al,[19] 2012	29	Chest wall restrictive	Prospective observational 3 months	No difference between masks in short-term or long-term gas exchange or adherence. 60% preferred NM.
Majorksi et al,[24] 2021	30	COPD	RXT, single night each arm	Tendency for improved sleep efficiency with ONM. SWS higher with ONM, with comparable mean $TcCO_2$ levels.
Lebret et al,[25] 2021	290	COPD and OHS	IPD and meta-analysis	86% of cases prescribed ONM. No difference between masks in daytime $Paco_2$, Pao_2, or adherence. IPAP was almost 2 cmH_2O higher with ONM. No interaction between primary pathology and mask type on outcome measures found.
Leotard et al,[23] 2021	30	NMD using NIV	RXT, 1 week each arm	No between group differences in primary outcome of mean nocturnal SpO_2, or secondary outcomes of %TST with SpO_2 <90%, ODI, level of unintentional leak or side effects. Changing masks affect NIV efficacy and increased reported side effects.

Abbreviations: AHI, apnea hypopnea index; COPD, chronic obstructive pulmonary disease; IPAP, inspiratory positive airway pressure; IPD, individual participant data; NIV, noninvasive ventilation; NMD, neuromuscular disease; NREM, non-rapid eye movement; ODI, oxygen desaturation index; OHS, obesity hypoventilation syndrome; ONM, oronasal mask; REM, rapid eye movement; RXT, randomized cross-over trial; SWS, slow wave sleep; TST, total sleep time.

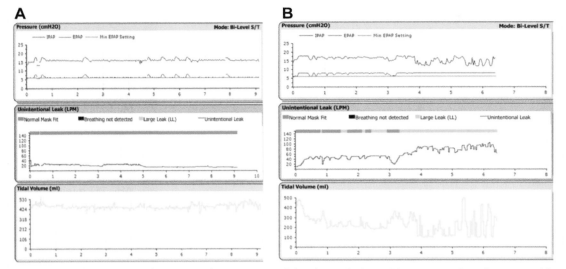

Fig. 4. Overnight summary download of a patient on bilevel ventilation with automated expiratory positive airway pressure (EPAP). (*A*) Unintentional leak is low throughout the night and set IPAP is maintained. (*B*) During a night of high unintentional leak, not only is tidal volume substantially lower, but the device is unable to maintain the set IPAP level.

may be severely compromised by frequent arousals in response to these events. High unintentional leak has also been associated with persistence of hypercapnia in neuromuscular conditions.[33]

Home ventilators now incorporate in-built software capable of providing data on various outputs such as leak and tidal volume.[34] Clinicians frequently use these data to identify potential issues with the efficacy of home NIV, triggering changes in care, including adjustment of ventilator settings if tidal volumes appear to be inappropriate.[13] However, several benchtop studies have demonstrated that the estimation of leak and tidal volume by in-built software can vary significantly depending on the intentional leak of mask used, pressure settings, and ventilator brand.[35,36] In addition, the software can underestimate[35,37] or overestimate[38,39] delivered tidal volumes depending on whether unintentional leaks are continuous or dynamic.[30] This is particularly relevant when using adaptive modes of ventilation, as the device may fail to deliver the preset tidal volume target due to inaccurate estimates of actual tidal volume delivery.[36,39,40]

For individuals using a nasal mask, the addition of a chinstrap may be sufficient to reduce leak and improve adherence.[20,41,42] Otherwise, a trial of an interface covering the mouth should be undertaken, with monitoring. If unsuccessful, inspiratory pressure may need to be reduced, with the goal of lessening leak and improving mask seal, although tidal volume may also decrease.

Dead Space

One of the risks proposed early on associated with using a mask and a single limb circuit was the potential for CO_2 rebreathing to compromise the effectiveness of NIV.[43] There were concerns that the larger inner volume of oronasal masks, representing additional dead space, could promote larger volumes of CO_2 being trapped within the mask and subsequently rebreathed. However, lung model studies[44,45] and a short-term clinical study[46] have shown that positioning the exhalation vents within the mask prevents CO_2 rebreathing by creating an advantageous flow pathway, which reduces dynamic dead space[45] and promotes CO_2 washout[46] (**Fig. 5**).

The intentional leak built into a vented mask is calibrated such that the degree of leak varies from mask brand and type,[47] as well as the level of pressure set.[27] However, if these vents become occluded, intentional leak will be reduced and increased levels of CO_2 may remain in the mask, permitting rebreathing. Issues with venting can occur intentionally when a user or carer blocks the vents to "reduce leak" or from poor cleaning practices allowing particulate matter to build up in the vents. Home ventilator users should be educated around the mask design and the role intentional leak plays in clearing CO_2 from the system.

Upper Airway Obstruction

One mechanism by which nasal continuous positive airway pressure (CPAP) works is through the

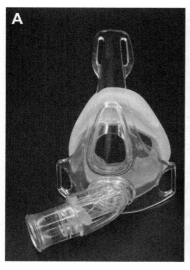 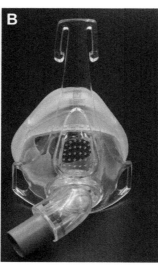

Fig. 5. Examples of non-vented (*A*) and vented (*B*) oronasal masks. Positioning of the exhalation vents within the mask itself promotes more efficient CO_2 clearance compared to placing the expiratory vents externally. (*Courtesy of* Dr Collette Menadue and Dr Kerri Melehan)

application of a splinting pressure in the posterior pharynx, helping push the tongue and the soft palate forward, thereby increasing the retropalatal cross-sectional area.[48] In contrast, with the application of positive pressure simultaneously in both the oral and nasal passages, this pressure gradient is lost, and the size of the retropalatal area is again reduced.[21] Several CPAP studies have shown that oronasal masks, by promoting oral breathing, encourage movement of the tongue and mandible posteriorly,[21,49,50] resulting in higher residual obstructive events.[51] The supine position[52] and rapid eye movement (REM) sleep further increase the likelihood of reduced upper airway dimensions.

Weakness of the tongue and pharyngeal muscles is common in people with neuromuscular conditions, which again favors upper airway obstruction occurring during sleep, especially in REM sleep and with the use of an oronasal mask.[53,54] Vrijsen and colleagues[55] demonstrated the possibility of the tongue being pushed backwards during inspiration with an oronasal mask, exacerbated by mouth opening under the mask. This could compromise ventilation and reduce sleep quality if machine pressures are not increased, potentially also affecting mask seal and comfort. Studies of patients with amyotrophic lateral sclerosis using home NIV have shown that those with persistence of upper airway obstruction on therapy experience shorter survival times compared to those more effectively ventilated,[56,57] even if nocturnal hypoxemia is not present.[56] Switching to a nasal mask may be effective, although a chinstrap is often needed to minimize mouth leak.[20,55,56] Overtightening of the lower

mask straps should be avoided as this can promote backward movement of the mandible, further reducing the oropharyngeal space. Changing the patient's position, especially moving them from lying supine, may also help. When other strategies fail, a reduction in IPAP may need to be considered.[55]

POTENTIAL MASK-ASSOCIATED COMPLICATIONS
Pressure Areas

Prolonged use of a mask, irrespective of the style or brand, can create significant damage to the skin and underlying tissues, particularly over the nasal bridge and cheeks[58] (**Fig. 6**). This damage arises from both compressive forces and shear stresses applied at points of contact between the skin and the mask cushion. Fitting an oronasal mask is often more difficult as it must cover more anatomic features simultaneously. In addition, the variability of mouth opening between wakefulness and different sleep stages can alter the distance between the nasion and the labiomental fold, causing slippage of the oronasal mask down the face. Certain patient characteristics such as age, steroid use, hypoxia, previous skin injury, and facial asymmetry may also increase the risk of skin damage.[26] While the pressure over the nasal bridge does not appear to increase with higher IPAP levels,[59] it can vary significantly between brands and styles of mask, as well as with body position.[59,60] Subjective reports of mask comfort are not considered sensitive enough to identify excessive nasal bridge pressure, especially in NIV-naïve individuals.[59]

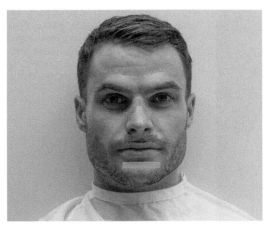

Fig. 6. Pressure areas with skin and tissue breakdown can develop at any point where the mask contacts the skin. However, the most common area where issues may arise is at the nasal bridge. Red areas indicate pressure contact points with nasal and oronasal masks. Tissue damage or pressure over the top of the upper lip can occur with nasal masks, pillows, and hybrid masks, indicated by the blue area. Oronasal and hybrid masks can apply additional pressure below the bottom lip, highlighted by the green line. Using a rotational mask strategy can reduce the risk of these injuries occurring. (*Courtesy of* Dr Collette Menadue and Dr Kerri Melehan)

Several approaches can be used to try and minimize this problem. Foremost is to ensure the mask style and brand chosen is of an appropriate size and fit. Overall, the pressure exerted on the face should be kept as low as possible, avoiding excessively tightening the headstraps. Regular care and replacement of the mask is important as wear and tear will alter the mechanical properties and integrity of the mask cushion. As pressure on the nasal bridge is less in the supine position compared to sitting,[59] it has also been suggested that mask fitting and headstrap adjustment be performed with the patient recumbent.[59] Rotation of different mask styles night-to-night or across the 24 hour period avoids constant pressure over the same area, reducing the risk of skin damage.

A wound dressing over the at-risk or reddened areas is often used to provide some protection and cushioning between of the mask and skin. Adhesive dressings are not recommended as they can be difficult to remove and can cause further skin damage during the removal process. Some mask cushions are now made of a memory foam which can conform more closely to the patient's facial features, reducing the pressure needed to maintain a seal.

Facial Side Effects

Changes in bone growth and formation can occur with long-term use of masks for positive airway pressure therapy, primarily in children,[61,62] although this may also occur in adults.[63] In an observational study of 40 children using masks for CPAP and NIV, Fauroux and colleagues[61] reported global facial flattening and maxillary retrusion in 68% and 37% of their cohort, respectively. Facial flattening was more commonly seen in patients with obstructive sleep apnea or a neuromuscular disorder, while maxillary retrusion was associated with using NIV more than 10 hours per day. Using cephalometric measurements in children prescribed CPAP, Roberts and colleagues[62] found those compliant with therapy experienced a significant degree of midface growth restriction compared to CPAP noncompliant children. Along with mask rotation, regular maxillofacial and orthodontic evaluations to allow early intervention are also recommended.[61,62]

Nasal Congestion and Oral Dryness

Large amounts of air passing across the nasal mucosa or open mouth can cause several problems including nasal congestion, oral dryness, or rhinitis. Minimizing leak and adding humidification can benefit some patients. For others, nasal saline washouts, corticosteroids, and anti-inflammatory medications should be considered.

Eye Irritation

Leak from the mask into the eyes can cause dryness and irritation of the eyes, increasing the risk of eye infections such as conjunctivitis.[64] Matossian and colleagues[65] examined the real-world incidence and prevalence of dry eye disease in people using CPAP for obstructive sleep apnea. Rates for both were significantly higher in those using CPAP for at least 36 months compared to the general population. The most direct solution is to refit the mask to avoid leakage into the eyes. Nasal prongs can often provide a good alternative, especially during daytime use. If the patient is unable to maintain a lip seal with a nasal mask, a hybrid style mask may offer an alternative to the standard oronasal mask. Prescription of lubricating eye drops and emollients has also been recommended.[64]

Claustrophobia

For many patients the idea of putting a mask over their face and then trying to sleep is a daunting prospect, triggering anxiety, and feelings of claustrophobia. In these situations, patience and trust needs to be developed between the clinician and the patient, ensuring the patient is educated and involved in the decision-making process. A slow introduction to use of the mask is needed, often starting with lower pressures and flow rates during wakefulness to help ease the patient into the sensations associated with mask use. Use of minimal contact masks such as nasal masks and pillows can often be less confronting than larger oronasal and full-face masks. Mouthpiece ventilation during daytime practise sessions can also be a useful introduction to therapy for some patients.[66]

SUMMARY

For most people requiring home NIV, therapy will be lifelong. For a smaller group, nocturnal therapy will eventually extend into continuous therapy use. As the link between the ventilator user and their "external respiratory pump," the interface is a crucial element in the acceptance, efficacy, and comfort of NIV support. While mask design, materials, and technology have improved over the past 40 years, there is still a long way to go in developing the "ideal" mask. Personalization of the interface is of particular importance for those individuals whose craniofacial features are outside the generalized norm catered for by currently available commercial masks. Although several randomized trials have failed to detect significant mean differences in outcomes among different mask styles, at an individual level clinical response and comfort can vary significantly. Despite increasing evidence around the impact of different interfaces for long-term home NIV, choosing the optimal interface in any given situation remains an art.

CLINICS CARE POINTS

- Reassessment of the efficacy of NIV should be undertaken when changing the style of interface.

- Oronasal masks can promote upper airway obstruction especially in the supine position and REM sleep.

- High unintentional leak from the interface can affect the efficacy and comfort of NIV with adverse impacts on ventilator performance.

- To reduce the risk of skin damage, rotating mask styles and designs is important for patients using NIV for extended daily periods or those with fragile skin.

ACKNOWLEDGMENTS

The author would like to thank Dr Collette Menadue and Dr Kerri Melehan for assistance in producing the photographs used in this article.

DISCLOSURE

The author reports income related to medical education conducted on behalf of ResMed and Philips, manufacturers of bilevel devices and interfaces for noninvasive ventilation.

REFERENCES

1. Pierucci P, Crimi C, Carlucci A, et al. Reinvent: ERS International survey on REstrictive thoracic diseases IN long term home noninvasive VENTilation. ERJ Open Res 2021;7:00911–2020.
2. Garner DJ, Berlowitz DJ, Douglas J, et al. Home mechanical ventilation in Australia and New Zealand. Eur Respir J 2013;41:39–45.
3. Callegari J, Magnet FS, Taubner S, et al. Interfaces and ventilator settings for long-term noninvasive ventilation in COPD patients. Int J Chronic Obstr Pulm Dis 2017;12:1883–9.
4. Crimi C, Noto A, Princi P, et al. Domiciliary noninvasive ventilation in COPD: an International survey of indications and practices. COPD 2016;13: 483–90.
5. Toussaint M, Chatwin M, Gonçalves MR, et al. Mouthpiece ventilation in neuromuscular disorders: narrative review of technical issues important for clinical success. Respir Med 2021;180:106373.
6. McDermott I, Bach JR, Parker C, et al. Custom-fabricated interfaces for intermittent positive pressure ventilation. Int J Prosthodont (IJP) 1989;2:224–33.
7. Duong K, Glover J, Perry AC, et al. Feasibility of three-dimensional facial imaging and printing for producing customised nasal masks for continuous positive airway pressure. ERJ Open Res 2021;7: 00632–2020.
8. Willox M, Metherall P, McCarthy AD, et al. Custom-made 3D printed masks for children using noninvasive ventilation: a comparison of 3D scanning technologies and specifications for future clinical service use, guided by patient and professional experience. J Med Eng Technol 2021;45:457–72.
9. Shikama M, Nakagami G, Noguchi H, et al. Development of personalized fitting device with 3-dimensional solution for prevention of NIV oronasal mask-related pressure ulcers. Respir Care 2018; 63:1024–32.
10. Lloyd-Owen SJ, Donaldson GC, Ambrosino N, et al. Patterns of home mechanical ventilation use in Europe: results from the Eurovent survey. Eur Respir J 2005;25:1025–31.

11. Navalesi P, Fanfulla F, Frigerio P, et al. Physiologic evaluation of noninvasive mechanical ventilation delivered with three types of masks in patients with chronic hypercapnic respiratory failure. Crit Care Med 2000;28:1785–90.

12. Teschler H, Stampa J, Ragette R, et al. Effect of mouth leak on effectiveness of nasal bilevel ventilatory assistance and sleep architecture. Eur Respir J 1999;14:1251–7.

13. Mansell SK, Cutts S, Hackney I, et al. Using domiciliary non-invasive ventilator data downloads to inform clinical decision-making to optimise ventilation delivery and patient compliance. BMJ Open Respir Res 2018;5:e000238.

14. Windisch W, Haenel M, Storre JH, et al. High-intensity non-invasive positive pressure ventilation for stable hypercapnic COPD. Int J Med Sci 2009;6:72–6.

15. Köhnlein T, Windisch W, Köhler D, et al. Non-invasive positive pressure ventilation for the treatment of severe stable chronic obstructive pulmonary disease: a prospective, multicentre, randomised, controlled clinical trial. Lancet Respir Med 2014;2:698–705.

16. Schwarz SB, Magnet FS, Windisch W. Why high-intensity NPPV is favourable to low-Intensity NPPV: clinical and physiological reasons. COPD 2017;14: 389–95.

17. Banfi P, Pierucci P, Volpato E, et al. Daytime noninvasive ventilatory support for patients with ventilatory pump failure: a narrative review. Multidiscip Respir Med 2019;14:38.

18. Bédard ME, McKim DA. Daytime mouthpiece for continuous noninvasive ventilation in individuals with amyotrophic lateral sclerosis. Respir Care 2016;61:1341–8.

19. Fernandez R, Cabrera C, Rubinos G, et al. Nasal versus oronasal mask in home mechanical ventilation: the preference of patients as a strategy for choosing the interface. Respir Care 2012;57:1413–7.

20. Willson GN, Piper AJ, Norman M, et al. Nasal versus full face mask for noninvasive ventilation in chronic respiratory failure. Eur Respir J 2004;23:605–9.

21. Andrade RG, Madeiro F, Genta PR, et al. Oronasal mask may compromise the efficacy of continuous positive airway pressure on OSA treatment: is there evidence for avoiding the oronasal route? Curr Opin Pulm Med 2016;22:555–62.

22. Masa JF, Utrabo I, Gomez de Terreros J, et al. Noninvasive ventilation for severely acidotic patients in respiratory intermediate care units: precision medicine in intermediate care units. BMC Pulm Med 2016;16:97.

23. Léotard A, Lebret M, Daabek N, et al. Impact of interface type on noninvasive ventilation efficacy in patients with neuromuscular disease: a randomized cross-over trial. Arch Bronconeumol 2021;57:273–80.

24. Majorski DS, Callegari JC, Schwarz SB, et al. Oronasal versus nasal masks for non-invasive ventilation in COPD: a randomized crossover trial. Int J Chronic Obstr Pulm Dis 2021;16:771–81.

25. Lebret M, Léotard A, Pépin JL, et al. Nasal versus oronasal masks for home non-invasive ventilation in patients with chronic hypercapnia: a systematic review and individual participant data meta-analysis. Thorax 2021;76:1108–16.

26. Brill A-K. How to avoid interface problems in acute noninvasive ventilation. Breath 2014;10:231–42.

27. Borel JC, Sabil A, Janssens JP, et al. Intentional leaks in industrial masks have a significant impact on efficacy of bilevel noninvasive ventilation: a bench test study. Chest 2009;135:669–77.

28. Louis B, Leroux K, Isabey D, et al. Effect of manufacturer-inserted mask leaks on ventilator performance. Eur Respir J 2010;35:627–36.

29. Martí S, Ferré A, Sampol G, et al. Sleep increases leaks and asynchronies during home noninvasive ventilation: a polysomnographic study. J Clin Sleep Med 2022;18:225–33.

30. Lebret M, Fresnel E, Prouvez N, et al. Responses of bilevel ventilators to unintentional leak: a bench study. Healthcare 2022;10:2416.

31. Al Otair HA, BaHammam AS. Ventilator- and interface-related factors influencing patient-ventilator asynchrony during noninvasive ventilation. Ann Thorac Med 2020;15:1–8.

32. Zhu K, Rabec C, Gonzalez-Bermejo J, et al. Combined effects of leaks, respiratory system properties and upper airway patency on the performance of home ventilators: a bench study. BMC Pulm Med 2017;17:145.

33. Gonzalez J, Sharshar T, Hart N, et al. Air leaks during mechanical ventilation as a cause of persistent hypercapnia in neuromuscular disorders. Intensive Care Med 2003;29:596–602.

34. Janssens JP, Borel JC, Pépin JL, et al. Nocturnal monitoring of home non-invasive ventilation: the contribution of simple tools such as pulse oximetry, capnography, built-in ventilator software and autonomic markers of sleep fragmentation. Thorax 2011;66:438–45.

35. Luján M, Sogo A, Pomares X, et al. Effect of leak and breathing pattern on the accuracy of tidal volume estimation by commercial home ventilators: a bench study. Respir Care 2013;58:770–7.

36. Luján M, Lalmolda C, Ergan B. Basic Concepts for tidal volume and leakage estimation in non-invasive ventilation. Turk Thorac J 2019;20:140–6.

37. Contal O, Vignaux L, Combescure C, et al. Monitoring of noninvasive ventilation by built-in software of home bilevel ventilators: a bench study. Chest 2012;141:469–76.

38. Sogo A, Montanyà J, Monsó E, et al. Effect of dynamic random leaks on the monitoring accuracy of home mechanical ventilators: a bench study. BMC Pulm Med 2013;13:75.

39. Luján M, Sogo A, Grimau C, et al. Influence of dynamic leaks in volume-targeted pressure support noninvasive ventilation: a bench study. Respir Care 2015;60:191–200.

40. Khirani S, Louis B, Leroux K, et al. Harms of unintentional leaks during volume targeted pressure support ventilation. Respir Med 2013;107:1021–9.

41. Knowles SR, O'Brien DT, Zhang S, et al. Effect of addition of chin strap on PAP compliance, nightly duration of use, and other factors. J Clin Sleep Med 2014;10:377–83.

42. Berry RB, Chediak A, Brown LK, et al. Best clinical practices for the sleep center adjustment of noninvasive positive pressure ventilation (NPPV) in stable chronic alveolar hypoventilation syndromes. J Clin Sleep Med 2010;6:491–509.

43. Lofaso F, Brochard L, Touchard D, et al. Evaluation of carbon dioxide rebreathing during pressure support ventilation with airway management system (Bi-PAP) devices. Chest 1995;108:772–8.

44. Schettino GP, Chatmongkolchart S, Hess DR, et al. Position of exhalation port and mask design affect CO_2 rebreathing during noninvasive positive pressure ventilation. Crit Care Med 2003;31:2178–82.

45. Saatci E, Miller DM, Stell IM, et al. Dynamic dead space in face masks used with noninvasive ventilators: a lung model study. Eur Respir J 2004;23:129–35.

46. Franke KJ, Schroeder M, Domanski U, et al. Noninvasive ventilation: effect of vented and non-vented exhalation systems on inspiratory CO_2 and O_2 concentrations, ventilation, and breathing pattern. Lung 2022;200:251–60.

47. Medrinal C, Prieur G, Contal O, et al. Non-invasive ventilation: evaluation of CO_2 washout by intentional leaking in three recent oronasal masks. a pilot study. Minerva Anestesiol 2015;81:526–32.

48. Sullivan CE, Issa FG, Berthon-Jones M, et al. Reversal of obstructive sleep apnoea by continuous positive airway pressure applied through the nares. Lancet 1981;1(8225):862–5.

49. Schorr F, Genta PR, Gregório MG, et al. Continuous positive airway pressure delivered by oronasal mask may not be effective for obstructive sleep apnoea. Eur Respir J 2012;40:503–5.

50. Ebben MR, Milrad S, Dyke JP, et al. Comparison of the upper airway dynamics of oronasal and nasal masks with positive airway pressure treatment using cine magnetic resonance imaging. Sleep Breath 2016;20:79–85.

51. Andrade RGS, Viana FM, Nascimento JA, et al. Nasal vs oronasal CPAP for OSA treatment: a meta-analysis. Chest 2018;153:665–74.

52. Nascimento JA, de Santana Carvalho T, Moriya HT, et al. Body position may influence oronasal CPAP effectiveness to treat OSA. J Clin Sleep Med 2016; 12:447–8.

53. Conde B, Martins N, Brandão M, et al. Upper Airway Video Endoscopy: assessment of the response to positive pressure ventilation and mechanical in-exsufflation. Pulmonology 2019;25:299–304.

54. Schellhas V, Glatz C, Beecken I, et al. Upper airway obstruction induced by non-invasive ventilation using an oronasal interface. Sleep Breath 2018;22:781–8.

55. Vrijsen B, Buyse B, Belge C, et al. Upper airway obstruction during noninvasive ventilation induced by the use of an oronasal mask. J Clin Sleep Med 2014;10:1033–5.

56. Georges M, Attali V, Golmard JL, et al. Reduced survival in patients with ALS with upper airway obstructive events on non-invasive ventilation. J Neurol Neurosurg Psychiatry 2016;87:1045–50.

57. Gonzalez-Bermejo J, Morelot-Panzini C, Arnol N, et al. Prognostic value of efficiently correcting nocturnal desaturations after one month of non-invasive ventilation in amyotrophic lateral sclerosis: a retrospective monocentre observational cohort study. Amyotroph Lateral Scler Frontotemporal Degener 2013;14:373–9.

58. Barros LS, Talaia P, Drummond M, et al. Facial pressure zones of an oronasal interface for noninvasive ventilation: a computer model analysis. J Bras Pneumol 2014;40:652–7.

59. Brill AK, Pickersgill R, Moghal M, et al. Mask pressure effects on the nasal bridge during short-term noninvasive ventilation. ERJ Open Res 2018;4:00168–2017.

60. Lin HL, Lee YC, Wang SH, et al. In vitro evaluation of facial pressure and air leak with a newly designed cushion for non-invasive ventilation masks. Healthcare 2020;8:523.

61. Fauroux B, Lavis JF, Nicot F, et al. Facial side effects during noninvasive positive pressure ventilation in children. Intensive Care Med 2005;31:965–9.

62. Roberts SD, Kapadia H, Greenlee G, et al. Midfacial and dental changes associated with nasal positive airway pressure in children with obstructive sleep apnea and craniofacial conditions. J Clin Sleep Med 2016;12:469–75.

63. Tsuda H, Almeida FR, Tsuda T, et al. Craniofacial changes after 2 years of nasal continuous positive airway pressure use in patients with obstructive sleep apnea. Chest 2010;138:870–4.

64. Shah PV, Zhu L, Kazi A, et al. The correlation between non-invasive ventilation use and the development of dry eye disease. Cureus 2021;13:e18280.

65. Matossian C, Song X, Chopra I, et al. The prevalence and incidence of dry eye disease among patients using continuous positive airway pressure or other nasal mask therapy devices to treat sleep apnea. Clin Ophthalmol 2020;14:3371–9.

66. Fiorentino G, Annunziata A, Cauteruccio R, et al. Mouthpiece ventilation in Duchenne muscular dystrophy: a rescue strategy for noncompliant patients. J Bras Pneumol 2016;42:453–6.

Telemonitoring in Non-invasive Ventilation

Sonia Khirani, PhD[a,b], Maxime Patout, MD[c,d], Jean-Michel Arnal, MD[e,*]

KEYWORDS

- Non-invasive ventilation • Continuous positive airway pressure • Telemonitoring
- Web-based platforms • Adult • Pediatrics • COPD • Neuromuscular disease

KEY POINTS

- Telemonitoring of home non-invasive ventilation (NIV) in adult and pediatric patients is attracting growing interest.
- Most ventilators are now equipped for telemonitoring and the various web-based platforms are constantly improving.
- Current solutions are aimed at monitoring daily use and leaks, whereas monitoring respiratory events and patient-ventilator synchrony requires more precise data and higher sample rates.
- Good coordination between homecare providers and hospital teams is needed to transform data into diagnosis, and action is a very important consideration.
- The main clinical benefits of telemonitoring comprise support of NIV initiation at home, improvement in the quality of NIV over time, and early detection of any deviation in order to decrease the risk of hospitalization.

INTRODUCTION

Telemonitoring of long-term home continuous positive airway pressure (CPAP) and non-invasive ventilation (NIV) for both adult and child care is attracting growing interest.[1–7] The recent coronavirus disease 2019 (COVID-19) pandemic has demonstrated its possible value as part of the management of patients on home CPAP/NIV.[3] Telemonitoring also represents a solution for overcoming the challenges of managing patients with chronic respiratory failure by: (1) delivering care to increasing numbers of adult and pediatric patients,[8] (2) improving long-term outcomes,[9] (3) improving care quality[10] with (4) limited healthcare resources, and (5) at a lower cost.[11]

Development of telemonitoring for long-term CPAP/NIV requires dedicated tools (communicating ventilators and platforms to access data), dedicated teams (home healthcare providers and hospital teams), and funding. With this support, efficiency of CPAP/NIV delivery may improve at treatment initiation and during long-term follow-up, allowing early detection of any worsening of the underlying respiratory condition.[12–14]

This review provides a summary of data available for telemonitoring in commonly used home ventilators and the web-based platforms used to access those data, while also addressing their limitations. It also discusses the potential management, clinical benefits, and clinical limitations of telemonitoring of CPAP/NIV. The focus is on adult

[a] ASV Santé, 125 Avenue Louis Roche, Gennevilliers 92230, France; [b] AP-HP Hôpital Necker-Enfants maladies, Unité de ventilation non-invasive et sommeil, 149 rue de Sèvres, Paris 75015, France; [c] AP-HP, Groupe Hospitalier Universitaire AP-HP-Sorbonne Université, site Pitié-Salpêtrière, Service des Pathologies du Sommeil (Département R3S), 47 Boulevard de l'hôpital, Paris 75013, France; [d] Sorbonne Université, INSERM, UMRS1158 Neurophysiologie Respiratoire Expérimentale et Clinique, Paris, France; [e] Service de Réanimation Polyvalente et Unité de Ventilation à Domicile, Hôpital Sainte Musse, Toulon 83100, France
* Corresponding author. Service de Réanimation Polyvalente et Unité de Ventilation à Domicile, Hôpital Sainte Musse, 54 rue Sainte Claire Deville, Toulon 83100, France.
E-mail address: jean-michel@arnal.org

Sleep Med Clin 19 (2024) 443–460
https://doi.org/10.1016/j.jsmc.2024.04.007
1556-407X/24/© 2024 Elsevier Inc. All rights reserved.

and pediatric NIV, as well as pediatric CPAP when performed using level 2 and level 3 ventilators.

THE TECHNICAL SOLUTIONS

In the section below, we review the technical features for telemonitoring with the different ventilators used for NIV in adult and pediatric patients, and for CPAP in children below 30 kg, as well as the data available on the different web-based platforms.

Ventilators, Data Transmission, and Platforms

Modern ventilators record many respiratory variables at a high sample rate that can be interpreted using dedicated built-in software. The accuracy of data varies according to the type of variable being monitored.[15] The precision of data regarding unintentional leaks, apnea-hypopnea index (AHI), and tidal volume (VT) may range from acceptable to poorly accurate,[16–19] often being more challenging in pediatrics.[20,21]

Currently, most ventilators are equipped with either built-in or external teletransmission systems, and enable telemonitoring via web-based platforms (**Table 1**).[1,15] Data are processed by the ventilator before being teletransmitted by means of either bluetooth or cellular connections. This has the consequence of precluding real-time monitoring of home CPAP/NIV, and limiting data quality, as the sample rate is lower compared to the data downloaded directly from the ventilator.[15]

Each manufacturer provides a specific web-based platform to display data from their own ventilators. Data vary greatly according to the ventilator, the modality of ventilation (CPAP or NIV), and the manufacturer. Web-based platforms that gather data from several manufacturers are also available (Vestalis Vision, Adel Santé), but the amount and detail of variables may be lower than that on the manufacturer's own web-based platform.

Telemonitored Variables

Data on CPAP/NIV usage, device pressures, system and mask leaks, respiratory rate (RR), VT, minute ventilation (MV), inspiratory (Ti) and expiratory (Te) times, triggered breaths, cycled breaths, and AHI are accessible on most web-based platforms (**Table 2**). Data are presented in the form of statistics, graphs, and trends. The telemonitored variables are measured from the ventilator's output. As the VT, RR, Ti, and Te may differ from the patient's physiologic variables, telemonitoring of NIV is valuable for following the treatment, rather than accurately assessing the patient's physiologic condition.

In young children, inadequate detection of the patient's airflow may be problematic. The telemonitored data may be inaccurate when the patient's airflow is not correctly detected by the ventilator,[20] resulting in some variables only being displayed intermittently or not at all, or displayed with inaccurate values, affecting the statistics and trends data. Moreover, as triggering and cycling may be not detected, statistics and trends for variables such as RR, Ti and the percentage of triggered and cycled breaths may also be affected.

Statistics

Statistics may either be partly available on the web-based platform and partly in a portable document format (pdf) report, or solely in the pdf report that needs to be created. The type of statistics provided (average, median, percentiles, maximum) vary according to the device and the web-based platform, while the way statistics are presented may differ from the built-in software for the same device. Statistics on usage and leaks may be helpful for following tolerance and efficacy of CPAP/NIV. Usage combines mean or median daily use and adherence, which details the timing of CPAP/NIV sessions, and the fragmentation of usage. Median unintentional leaks below 10 to 12 L/min and 95th percentile below 20 to 24 L/min are commonly accepted,[15,19] although low levels of leaks have been associated with poorer sleep quality.[22] In addition to the level of leakage, a bench study has demonstrated that the pattern of leakage (intermittent leaks) appears to have more impact on the device performance and patient-ventilator asynchronies than does the magnitude of the leak flow rate itself.[23] This highlights the fact that overnight trend data may be more useful than statistical values.

Measurements of time, such as Ti and Te, inspiratory:expiratory (I:E) ratio, and the percentage of spontaneous triggering and cycling, are generally considered accurate. RR should be interpreted as the ventilatory rate, and may therefore not always correspond with the patient's RR. Statistical values for VT, MV and AHI should also be interpreted with caution due to their lack of accuracy, especially in the presence of unintentional leaks.[16,18,21,24] However, in the absence of unintentional leaks, a low VT can be considered correct and should be acted upon.

In contrast, in children a low VT or the absence of VT values may in some cases be an indication of difficulties with detection of the patient's airflow.[20] Furthermore, statistical values for AHI should be considered with greater caution in children, due to an inadequate scoring of respiratory events by the device.[21]

Table 1
Web-based platforms for CPAP/NIV telemonitoring

Web-based Platform	Devices	Connectivity	Data Transmission	Daily Trend Data	Overnight Trend	Clinical Alerts	Remote Settings	External Monitors
Airview (ResMed)	Lumis	Cellular internal	Daily, 1 h following NIV stop, with device on standby	Yes	Yes (1 point/min)	Yes (AirView Ventilation Expert)	Yes	SpO_2
Airview (ResMed)	Stellar, Astral	Cellular external	Daily from 12 PM if device turned on (with power supply or on internal battery), with NIV running or not and module connected	Yes	Yes (1 point/min)	Yes (AirView Ventilation expert)	No	SpO_2
Care Orchestrator (Philips Respironics)	DreamStation BiPAP, BiPAP A30, BiPAP A40 pro, BiPAP A40 EFL	PR1 cellular modem	Daily	Yes	Yes (1 point/2 min)	Yes	Yes	SpO_2, HR
Care Orchestrator (Philips Respironics)	Trilogy 100/200, Trilogy Evo	Bluetooth cellular hub	Every 8 h	Yes	Yes (1 point/5 min)	Yes	No	SpO_2, HR, Fio_2, ($PetCO_2$?)[a]
EveryWare (Breas Medical)	Vivo 1-2-3, Vivo 45/45LS, Nippy 4	Cellular external	Every 15 min	Yes	Yes (1 point/breath)	Yes	Yes	SpO_2, $PetCO_2$, $PtCO_2$
PrismaCLOUD (Löwenstein)	prisma25ST, prisma30ST, prismaVENT 30-C, 40, 50, 50-C	Cellular external	Twice a day	Yes (usage and leaks; other variable on pdf report)	Only on pdf report (1 point/2 min)	No	Yes	SpO_2, HR
Vestalis vision (Air Liquide)	EO-150	Cellular internal 4G	Daily	Yes	Only by download	Yes	No	SpO_2, HR, $PtCO_2$

Abbreviations: HR, heart rate; $PetCO_2$, partial pressure of end-tidal carbon dioxide; $PtCO_2$, transcutaneous carbon dioxide; SpO_2, pulse oximetry.
[a] Telemonitoring will be available on a short term.

Table 2
Variables monitored on the different web-based platforms

Web-based Platform	Daily Usage	Leaks	AHI	Synchronization	Other Variables	SpO₂ HR	PetCO₂ PtcCO₂
Airview (ResMed)	*Daily trend* usage, fragmentation (rolling 90 d max) *Statistics* (rolling 90 d max) *Overnight trend* (zoom max: 1h, 1 pt/min)	*Daily trend* (rolling 90 d max) *Statistics* (rolling 90 d max) *Overnight trend* (zoom max: 1h, 1 pt/min)	*Daily trend* (rolling 90 d max) *Statistics* (rolling 90 d max) *Overnight trend* (zoom max: 1h, 1 pt/min)	*Daily trend* % spontaneous trigger and cycle (rolling 90 d max) *Statistics* % spontaneous trigger and cycle (rolling 90 d max) *Overnight trend* % spontaneous trigger and cycle (zoom max: 1h, 1 pt/min)	*Daily trend* IPAP, EPAP, VT, RR, MV, I:E ratio, Ti, RSBI (rolling 90 d max) *Statistics* IPAP, EPAP, VT, RR, MV, I:E ratio, Ti, Te, RSBI, max inspiratory flow (rolling 90 d max) *Overnight trend* IPAP, EPAP, VT, RR, MV, I:E ratio, Ti, Te, RSBI (zoom max: 1h, 1 pt/min)	*Daily trend* SpO₂ (rolling 90 d max) *Statistics* SpO₂ (rolling 90 d max) *Overnight trend* SpO₂ (zoom max: 1h, 1 pt/min)	No
Care Orchestrator (Philips Respironics)	*Daily trend* usage, fragmentation (adjustable period) *Statistics* (adjustable period) *Overnight trend* (adjustable period) (1 pt/2 or 5 min)	*Daily trend on pdf report* (adjustable period) *Statistics* (adjustable period) *Overnight trend on pdf report* (adjustable period) (1 pt/2 or 5 min)	*Daily trend on pdf report* (adjustable period) *Statistics* (adjustable period) *Overnight trend* (adjustable period) (1 pt/2 or 5 min)	*Daily trend on pdf report* % spontaneous trigger (adjustable period) *Statistics on pdf report* % spontaneous trigger (adjustable period) *Overnight trend on pdf report* % spontaneous trigger (adjustable period) (1 pt/2 or 5 min)	*Daily trend on pdf report* IPAP, EPAP, VT, RR, MV, Ti/Ttot (adjustable period) *Statistics* IPAP, VT, RR, MV (adjustable period) *Overnight trend on pdf report* IPAP, EPAP, VT, RR, MV, Ti/Ttot, alarms (adjustable period)	*Daily trend* SpO₂, HR (adjustable period) *Statistics* SpO₂, HR (adjustable period) *Overnight trend* SpO₂, HR (adjustable period) (1 pt/2 or 5 min)	No

(1 pt/2 or 5 min)

EveryWare (Breas Medical)	Daily trend usage (over 30 d adjustable) Statistics usage (over 30 d adjustable)	Daily trend (over 30 d adjustable) Statistics (over 30 d adjustable) Overnight trend (zoom max: 5 min, 1 pt/5 s)	Statistics (over 30 d adjustable)	Breath by breath waveforms on pdf report[a] airway pressure and airflow (adjustable period) (6 min per line) Daily trend IPAP, EPAP, VT (over 30 d adjustable) Statistics EPAP, Ppeak, VT (over 30 d adjustable) Overnight trend IPAP, EPAP, VT, RR (zoom max: 5 min, 1 pt/5 s)	Overnight trend SpO$_2$, HR (zoom max: 5 min, 1 pt/5 s)	Overnight trend PetCO$_2$, PtcCO$_2$ (zoom max: 5 min, 1 pt/5 s)
PrismaCLOUD (Löwenstein)	Daily trend Usage over 8 d, usage, and fragmentation on pdf report with adjustable period Statistics Usage over 8 d, usage on pdf with adjustable period Overnight trend on pdf report (1 pt/2 min)	Daily trend Over 8 d and on pdf report with adjustable period Statistics Over 8 d and on pdf report with adjustable period Overnight trend on pdf report (1 pt/2 min)	Daily trend Over 8 d and on pdf report with adjustable period Statistics Over 8 d and on pdf report with adjustable period Overnight trend on	Statistics % spontaneous trigger over 8 d and on pdf report with adjustable period Overnight trend on pdf report % spontaneous trigger and cycle (1 pt/2 min)	Daily trend on pdf report IPAP, EPAP, VT, RR (adjustable period) Statistics VT, RR, MV, Ti, Ti/Ttot over 8 d and on pdf report with adjustable period Overnight trend on pdf report IPAP, EPAP, VT, RR,	Statistics on pdf report Overnight trend on pdf report (1 pt/2 min)	No

(continued on next page)

Table 2
(continued)

Web-based Platform	Daily Usage	Leaks	AHI	Synchronization	Other Variables	SpO₂ HR	PetCO₂ PtcCO₂
Vestalis vision (Air Liquide)	*Daily trend* usage (over 365 d adjustable) *Statistics* (median and 95th; rolling 365 d max) *Overnight trend* by download	*Daily trend* usage (over 365 d adjustable) *Statistics* (median and 95th; rolling 365 d max) *Overnight trend* by download *Breath by breath waveforms* by download (zoom max: 10/5 s, 12/24 pt/sec)	*pdf report* (1 pt/2 min) *Breath by breath waveforms by download* (zoom max: 10/5 s, 12/24 pt/sec)	*Daily trend* % spontaneous trigger and cycle (rolling 365 d max) *Statistics* % spontaneous trigger and cycle (median and 95th; rolling 365 d max) *Overnight trend by download* % spontaneous trigger and cycle	MV, Ti/Ttot (1 pt/2 min) *Daily trend* IPAP, EPAP, VT, RR, MV, I:E ratio, Ti, VTi/VTe (rolling 365 d max) *Statistics* IPAP, EPAP, VT, RR, MV, I:E ratio, Ti, VTi/VTe (median and 95th; rolling 365 d max) *Overnight trend by download* IPAP, EPAP, VT, RR, MV, I:E ratio, Ti, VTi/VTe *Breath by breath waveforms by download* air pressure and flow, RR, VTi/VTe (zoom max: 10/5 s, 12/24 pt/sec)	*Overnight trend by download* *Breath by breath waveforms by download* (zoom max: 10/5 s, 12/24 pt/sec)	*Overnight trend by download* *Breath by breath waveforms by download* raw PtcCO₂, corrected PetCO₂, PtcCO₂ (zoom max: 10/5 s, 12/24 pt/sec)

Abbreviations: AHI, apnea-hypopnea index; EPAP, expiratory positive airway pressure; HR, heart rate; I:E ratio, inspiratory to expiratory ratio; IPAP, inspiratory positive airway pressure; MV, minute ventilation; PetCO₂, partial pressure of end-tidal carbon dioxide; Ppeak, peak pressure; PtcCO₂, transcutaneous carbon dioxide; RR, respiratory rate; RSBI, rapid and shallow breathing index; SpO₂, pulse oximetry; Te, expiratory time; Ti, inspiratory time; Ttot, total breath time; VT, tidal volume; VTe, expiratory tidal volume; VTi, inspiratory tidal volume.

[a] Except for BiPAP A30 and Trilogy Evo.

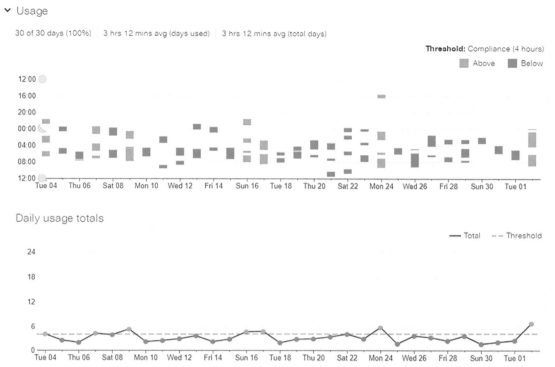

Fig. 1. Telemonitored trend usage of NIV in an adult patient. Upper panel: Daily usage over a 30-day period with the display of timing (Airview, ResMed). Note the intermittent usage with repeated interruptions to NIV during the sleep time. The red rectangles indicate usage of less than 4 hours/day. Bottom panel: Daily usage duration. Note that the patient mostly used NIV for less than 4 hours/day within the 1-month period.

Trends

The trend data available on web-based platforms are usually the same as the trend data available from the built-in software of the device. The number of days of data available to review on these platforms varies according to the device and manufacturer.

Usage data are normally displayed as the total daily use and the timing of use each day.[25] Thus, intermittent use across the whole night is visible (**Fig. 1**). Irregular or increased use of CPAP/NIV indicates a need to review the patient for the different possible causes.[1,2,26,27] Data regarding leaks are usually available from the ventilator's built-in software, including total leaks, unintentional leaks, or both. Although RR, VT, MV, and AHI data may not be accurate, a review of the trend of this data may be useful to help exclude clinical deterioration.[13,14,28]

Overnight trends may be very helpful for identifying major issues during the night, even though the data are displayed at low sample rates. Excessive leaks and, most importantly, the pattern of the leaks are valuable data for determining a suitable intervention depending on the cause of the leak (eg, mouth breathing, leaks due to a poorly fitting mask) (**Fig. 2**). Trend data in children may be inaccurate, with shorter reported usage data possibly due to a failure of the device to detect breathing (**Fig. 3**). On the overnight trends, intermittent measurements suggest improper detection of the patient's airflow.

Nocturnal recordings

The availability of home nocturnal pulse oximetry (SpO_2) and transcutaneous carbon dioxide ($PtcCO_2$) recording together with ventilator data may enable enhanced CPAP/NIV monitoring.[29] Nocturnal SpO_2 can provide a simple, low-cost screening tool to assess CPAP/NIV efficiency, and can be recorded using a stand-alone device or a sensor connected to the ventilator. This allows a visual review of the SpO_2 measurement within the built-in device software, in addition to information on unintentional leaks, pressure, and airflow waveforms. Currently, telemonitoring of nocturnal SpO_2 is possible, but sampling rates prevent the detection of some episodes of desaturation (**Fig. 4**).[15] Overnight $PtcCO_2$ monitoring combined with SpO_2 is essential, as a normal SpO_2 is not necessarily indicative of effective ventilation.[29,30] $PtcCO_2$ is usually measured using a stand-alone

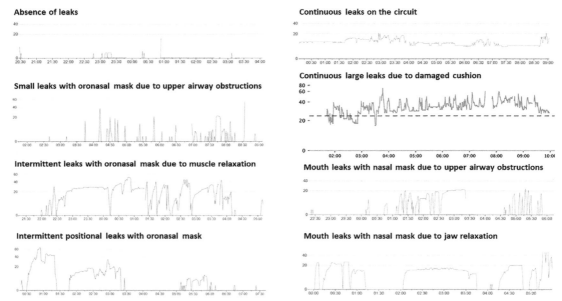

Fig. 2. Overnight trend data for unintentional leaks. Telemonitored overnight trends for unintentional leaks differ according to the mechanism of leakage. This information is useful for the telemonitoring team to help patients better manage leaks remotely.

capnograph. It is possible to connect the capnograph to some ventilators, so that measurements can be displayed by the built-in software. However, only one web-based platform is currently able to directly display $PtcCO_2$ data. Some $PtcCO_2$ devices require calibration of the sensor once the recording ends, in order to correct for drift in $PtcCO_2$ measurement that occurs over time. The data recorded by the built-in software and displayed on a web-based platform are therefore raw $PtcCO_2$ data with no drift correction.

What is missing?

Aside from web-based platforms still being "a work in progress", a number of issues can limit the use of telemonitoring for following patients on home CPAP/NIV. First, CPAP/NIV devices can be categorized in 3 levels. Level 1 NIV devices have no internal battery but an optional integrated heated humidifier. Level 2 devices have variable internal battery duration and optional integrated heated humidifiers. Level 3 devices—which are life support ventilators—must guarantee minimal battery

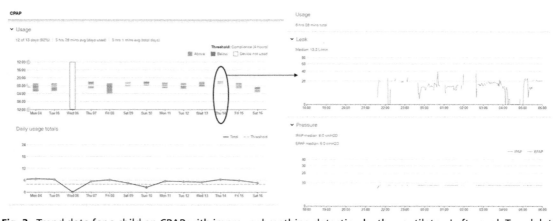

Fig. 3. Trend data for a child on CPAP with improper breathing detection by the ventilator. Left panel: Trend data for usage. Note the several interruptions to usage during the nights, and the discrepancies between the totals for fragmentation usage and daily usage. Right panel: Note the intermittent tracings display and the time discrepancy with the fragmentation usage and daily usage displayed on the left panel. The patient used the device for about 8 hours and not 6 ½ hours as reported. Airview web-based platform (ResMed).

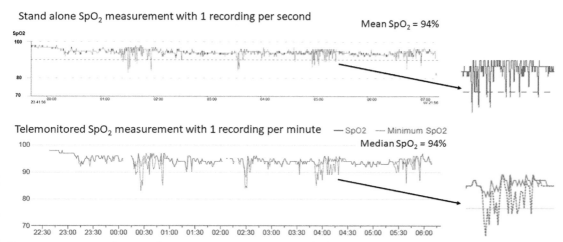

Fig. 4. Comparison of overnight SpO_2 measurement using a high-granularity standalone device and telemonitored SpO_2. Upper panel: SpO_2 measured by a Nonin device at 1 point per second. Bottom panel: SpO_2 measured with the sensor connected to a Lumis ventilator (ResMed) and telemonitored on Airview (ResMed) at 1 point per minute. Note that the median value reported on the web-based platform is in agreement with the mean value calculated by the standalone device. Trends are parallel for slow changes of SpO_2. Rapid changes of SpO_2 suggesting upper airway obstructions are demonstrated on the telemonitored trend by a difference between SpO_2 (*solid blue line*) and minimum SpO_2 (*dotted purple line*). Abbreviations: SpO_2, pulse oximetry.

duration of 8 hours, and have no internal heated humidifiers. Most level 1 and level 2 CPAP/NIV devices are already remotely accessible, in contrast to some level 3 devices. Although children may be treated with CPAP using a level 3 ventilator,[31] these may not be accessible for telemonitoring. Second, some web-based platforms provide ventilator data only on pdf reports, which may limit usability. Third, detailed breath-by-breath measurements are not available on most web-based platforms. Fourth, some ventilators offer modules to directly connect thoraco-abdominal belts and SpO_2/$PtcCO_2$ monitoring to the ventilator. Integrating these measurements in the built-in device software allows better characterization of residual events. However, as with sleep studies, the inability to view the recordings from the thoraco-abdominal belts on any web-based platform limits their utility for home follow-up. Finally, the web-based platforms do not allow the integration of patient information, such as patient-reported symptoms and experience measures.

Alerts

Alerts are intended for the automatic detection of significant deviations in telemonitored variables, and can be set up on the majority of web-based platforms. These represent the first step in transforming data into information that can support the telemonitoring team (homecare providers and healthcare professionals). The capabilities of alerts vary according to the different platforms; some of these incorporate fixed alerts, while others allow for the individualization of alerts (**Table 3**). Adequate threshold settings are necessary to avoid an excessive number of alerts. In pediatrics, it is important to ensure the patient's breathing is being detected correctly before setting alert thresholds, so as to avoid an excessive number of false alerts. A recent prospective observational study found that the day-to-day variability of monitored variables, over a period of 5 days, was much larger between clinically stable individuals using NIV at home for different diagnoses than within the group.[32] In addition, daily use, leaks, and AHI varied relatively more within participants than did VT, MV, RR, and the percentage of triggered breaths. To date, no study has evaluated the clinical benefits of using alerts. Nevertheless, alerts for independent variables such as daily use, leaks, AHI, and RR are of interest because any significant deviation may be informative. In contrast, dependent variables such as VT, MV, the percentage of triggered and cycled breaths, and the I:E ratio are less helpful because any deviation is usually the consequence of leaks or asynchrony. Therefore, the optimal setting and individualization of alerts is the key to efficient telemonitoring of CPAP/NIV.

Remote Adjustment of Ventilator Settings

When homecare providers and/or healthcare professionals telemonitor CPAP/NIV, they may detect more problems than are identified with conventional clinic reviews. However, telemonitored

Table 3
Alert capabilities of the web-based platforms

Web Based Platform	Transmission Alert	Utilization Alerts	Leaks Alert	Respiratory Events Alerts	RR Alerts	Other Alerts
Airview	Number of days without data transmission	Daily use threshold and number of consecutive days	Unintentional leaks threshold and number of consecutive days	AHI threshold and number of consecutive days	Minimum and maximum threshold and number of consecutive days, and deviation from the median value of the last 90 d	SpO₂ percentage of triggered breath, percentage of cycled breath, MV, VT
Care Orchestrator	Number of days without data transmission (Only if there is no transmission in the days following the device assignment)	Daily use threshold and number of consecutive days	Unintentional leaks threshold and number of days over a certain period Percentage of time with large leaks and number of days over a certain period	AHI threshold and number of days over a certain period Central apnea threshold and number of days over a certain period	Minimum and maximum threshold and number of consecutive days and deviation from mean value over a certain period	Percentage of time with periodic breathing and number of days over a certain period. Percentage of time with IPAP at maximum tolerated value and number of days over a certain period Ti/Ttot threshold and number of consecutive days, and variation of Ti/Tot. % inspiratory trigger and variation in % inspiratory trigger VT threshold and variation of VT. MV threshold and variation of MV

Breas EveryWare	Fixed alert: no transmission for 3 consecutive days	Daily use threshold for 3 consecutive days	None	None	None	Alert generated if a high priority alarm occurred at least 10 times within 24 h, or a high priority alarm lasted more than 5 min
PrismaCLOUD	None	None	None	None	None	None
Vestalis vision	Number of days without data transmission	Daily use threshold and number of consecutive days Daily use variation and number of days over 7 d	Unintentional leaks threshold and number of days over a certain period Leaks variation and number of days over 7 d	AHI threshold and number of days over a certain period AHI variation and number of days over 7 d	RR threshold and number of consecutive days over a certain period RR variation and number of days over 7 d	None

Settings that are adjustable by the user are underlined.

Abbreviations: AHI, apnea-hypopnea index; IPAP, inspiratory positive airway pressure; MV, minute volume; RR, respiratory rate; SpO_2, pulse oximetry; TI, inspiratory time; Ttot, total breath time; VT, tidal volume.

data alone are rarely sufficient to make a diagnosis, as this requires combining this data with symptoms reported by the patient. Measures required to improve the tolerance and/or efficiency of CPAP/NIV include either a change of interface, adjustment of ventilator settings, or the reinforcement of therapeutic education, according to the patient's circumstances. Telemonitoring of CPAP/NIV may lead to minor adjustments to ventilator settings that can be made remotely. Remote adjustment of ventilator settings is therefore complementary to telemonitoring. Technically, remote adjustments are only possible using the web-based platform designed by the ventilator's manufacturer. Currently, there are several ventilators offering remote adjustment of ventilation mode and settings, alarms, and the heated humidifier (**Table 4**). To prevent the inappropriate use of remote setting changes, it is necessary to define rules and criteria within the telemonitoring team (**Fig. 5**). Web-based platforms keep a record of remote adjustments showing the date and time, the setting adjusted, and the name of the clinician. While there is no published evidence on the use and utility of remote adjustments, this approach can be clinically useful when initiating NIV, for instance to progressively increase inspiratory positive airway pressure (IPAP) or adjust the synchronization settings.

Cost and Reimbursement

The cost of telemonitoring differs from country to country, and from manufacturer to manufacturer. Hardware costs may be included in the price of the ventilator device if it contains an internal cellular module. Additional costs may be incurred if an external cellular module is required. In addition, there may be a cost incurred to access the web-based platform, particularly if the platform is provided by an external company that can display data from several manufacturers. Furthermore, reimbursement of telemonitoring activity for CPAP/NIV is currently not available in all countries.[33]

COORDINATION

The entire telemonitoring process, starting from data collection through to medical decision-making, relies on a well-coordinated approach between the different stakeholders to ensure efficiency and optimal patient outcomes.[33]

The Telemonitoring Team

The patient is the major stakeholder in the telemonitoring team and, as such, patients need to be as actively involved as possible. Providing the patient or their caregiver with simplified but comprehensive information directly on the ventilator screen or through an application on their smartphone may help improve the quality of CPAP/NIV usage. To date, there are no self-management solutions available for NIV, but these seem likely to develop rapidly. Most patients are familiar with new technologies and ask for more information about their treatment. However, the introduction of NIV and telemonitoring can be a source of additional stress for some patients. Daily usage and unintentional leaks are the most important data to provide, because the patient or their caregiver can often manage these problems themselves. Trends for daily usage can help the patient achieve the clinician-set target. The benefits of adherence have been demonstrated in patients with obstructive sleep apnea using CPAP.[34–36] As leaks are often due to incorrect adjustment of the headgear and positioning of the mask, patients or caregivers can correct these problems themselves and monitor the effect. They may then seek support from the homecare providers if the problem persists. Conversely, providing too much information that the patient or caregiver cannot control, such as RR, AHI, and VT, may induce unnecessary anxiety.

Technicians working for homecare providers can support the telemonitoring program by checking the correct transmission of ventilator data and creating reports. With proper training and written protocols, they can also monitor the daily usage and leaks, and contact the patient to reinforce education. All other variables require medical knowledge to be interpreted and corrected. However, technicians can monitor those variables and alert clinicians in case of deviations.

Healthcare professionals such as nurses, physiotherapists, or respiratory therapists play a major role in telemonitoring. They can regularly review the data and alerts automatically generated by the platform and determine when a deviation is clinically significant. They can then contact the patient and link the ventilator data to the clinical symptoms using direct questioning or standardized questionnaires,[37–39] to determine if any action is required. That action may range from reinforcement of the patient's education to medical advice in the case of an adjustment to ventilator settings or suspicion of an acute exacerbation.

Physicians and nurse practitioners have overall responsibility for the telemonitoring program. They coordinate activities and design protocols and communication tools for the team. They may not necessarily be involved in the systematic review of ventilator data, but they should act as an advisor to support the team when needed, deciding on adjustments to ventilator settings or be available for consultation if an acute exacerbation is suspected.

Table 4
Capabilities of the different ventilators and web-based platforms to remotely change the ventilator settings

Web-based Platform	Ventilator	Ventilation Mode	EPAP/IPAP	Inspiratory Trigger and Cycling	Pressure Rise Time	Backup RR	Other
Airview	Lumis	Yes	Yes	Yes	Yes	Yes	Ramp time, min Ti, max Ti, humidification setting
Care Orchestrator	Dream Station BiPAP, BiPAP A30, BiPAP A40 pro, BiPAP A40 EFL	Yes	Yes	Yes (except for DreamStation)	Yes	Yes	Target VT, ramp time, backup Ti, alarms, humidification setting, mask type
Care Orchestrator	Trilogy 100/200, Trilogy Evo	No	No	No	No	No	No
Breas EveryWare	Vivo 1-2-3, Vivo 45, Nippy 4	Yes	Yes	Yes	Yes	Yes	Target VT, ramp time, min Ti, max Ti, backup Ti, alarms, humidification setting
PrismaCLOUD	prisma25ST, prisma30ST, prismaVENT 30-C, prismaVENT 40, prismaVENT 50, prismaVENT 50-C	Yes	Yes	Yes	Yes	Yes	Target VT, ramp time, min Ti, max Ti, backup Ti, soft start and soft stop, auto start and stop, alarms, humidification setting
Vestalis vision	EO 150	No	No	No	No	No	No

Abbreviations: EPAP, expiratory positive airway pressure; IPAP, inspiratory positive airway pressure; RR, respiratory rate; VT, tidal volume; Ti, inspiratory time.

- Define setting adjustment responsibilities:
  - EPAP, IPAP, and RR setting decided by physician, RT, physiotherapist, or NP
  - Other setting can be decided by trained nurses or technicians
- Remote ventilator settings are restricted to stable patients
- Ventilator setting change restricted to patient able to express discomfort
- Inform patient of the setting change
- Ask patient to test the new setting during daytime
- Provide a way to contact the telemonitoring team
- Monitor the outcome of the ventilator adjustment on subsequent days

Fig. 5. Example of rules defined within the telemonitoring team regarding the use of remote adjustment of ventilator settings. Abbreviations: EPAP, expiratory positive airway pressure; IPAP, inspiratory positive airway pressure; RR, respiratory rate; RT, respiratory therapist; NP, nurse practitioner.

Roles and activities of health professionals and physician/nurse practitioners can be interchangeable depending of the overall organization at each institution.

Possible Approaches to Implementing Telemonitoring

One possible approach to using telemonitoring involves technicians or healthcare professionals regularly screening the patient's daily usage data, leaks and AHI. Some platforms have designed a simplified display of this information with color-coding to help the reviewer rapidly screen potential issues (**Fig. 6**). These displays help the reviewer to focus on patients with abnormalities who then require a more detailed review of their data in order to determine the appropriate action.

Another possible approach is on-demand management triggered by alerts. In this case, the clinicians set some alerts to automatically detect deviations in the main variables, thereby prioritizing patients when an alert is generated. In general, the setting of appropriate alert thresholds that are sensitive and specific enough for clinically significant deviations to be detected remains a challenge for clinicians. If the alert is set too close to the patient's normal variability, it will generate repeated alerts that serve no purpose, but still take time to be analyzed by the telemonitoring team. Conversely, if the alert is set too far from the patient's normal variability, significant clinical events may go

Name	Days monitored	Mean daily use	27/07	28/07	29/07	30/07	31/07	01/08	02/08	03/08	04/08	05/08
MARYSE	17	4h 54m										
MOHAMED	21	5h 48m										
CHRISTINE	49	10h 53m										
MARCEL	62	4h 33m										
ANNE MARIE	76	7h 57m										
ANTOINE	82	7h 55m										
CHANTAL	83	4h 53m										
BERNARD	87	2h 34m										
JEANINE	110	6h 1m										
MARIE CHRISTINE	115	5h 31m										

Fig. 6. An example of the screening panel on the Airview platform (ResMed). Each line is for one patient. The square displays the daily use for the last 10 days. The green square is for daily use of more than 4 hours, the red square for less than 4 hours, and the white square if NIV was not used at all. The yellow line in the upper part of the square indicates large unintentional leaks. The yellow line in the lower part of the square indicates a high apnea-hypopnea index.

unnoticed. It seems possible that artificial intelligence technology will help to determine the appropriate settings and assist with analyzing variables to trigger alerts for specific events.

The optimal frequency for screening telemonitored variables or managing alerts remains unknown. Because respiratory failure can occur within days after NIV discontinuation,[40] reviewing telemonitored variables twice weekly would seem reasonable.

CLINICAL APPLICATION AND EVIDENCE

Because telemonitoring of NIV is relatively new, there is little clinical evidence and most published studies are observational with no control group.

Initiation of Non-Invasive Ventilation at Home

Telemonitoring of NIV is particularly useful when NIV is initiated at home, allowing the monitoring of patients closely during the first days of use, and to guide adjustments to ventilator settings.[41] A retrospective study compared in-hospital versus at-home initiation of NIV for patients with amyotrophic lateral sclerosis (ALS).[42] Initiation at home was performed by a specialist physiotherapist, who combined physical visits at home with telemonitoring. The delay between NIV prescription and initiation was much shorter and the daily use of NIV at 30 days after initiation was greater for patients initiating treatment at home.

Three randomized controlled trials have compared in-hospital versus at-home initiation of NIV supported by telemonitoring in chronic obstructive pulmonary disease (COPD), neuromuscular disease (NMD) (including patients with ALS), and chest wall restriction.[43–45] NIV was initiated at home by a specialist nurse, who then used telemonitoring and phone advice for subsequent management. $PtcCO_2$ monitoring was also performed several times at home. Ventilator settings were adjusted remotely when required. All studies reported that home initiation was non-inferior to hospital initiation in relation to improvement in daytime arterial carbon dioxide pressure and health-related quality of life. Limitations of these randomized clinical trials included the significant travel time for healthcare workers versus the high cost of in-hospital NIV initiation, compared to the costs incurred in ambulatory NIV initiation.[46]

Long-Term Telemonitoring After the Initiation Period

One potential clinical benefit of telemonitoring NIV is improving the quality of treatment by detecting deviations earlier and providing the appropriate support for the patient. An observational study including 329 adult patients with different lung conditions reported the benefits of telemonitoring of NIV over 12 months using automated alerts.[47] Alerts were managed by nurses working for the homecare provider, who also provided remote therapeutic education sessions. The proportion of patients meeting the criteria for successful NIV usage (daily usage >4h, median unintentional leak <24 L/min, and AHI <10/h) increased from 75% at inclusion to 86% at 6 months. In all patients, daily NIV use increased significantly over time and AHI significantly decreased, while unintentional leaks remained low during the entire period. The authors suggested that telemonitoring of NIV combined with therapeutic education was feasible and may be beneficial for patients. Interestingly, the alert management burden was 4.9 alerts per patient on average during the first 6 months and remained stable thereafter.

A recent case-controlled study compared the incidence and duration of hospitalization between telemonitored and non-telemonitored children with NMD ventilated at home by mask or tracheostomy.[7] Telemonitoring consisted of a weekly review of ventilator data with a recording of nocturnal SpO_2, followed by a weekly telephone call with the patient and family. Unscheduled calls from parents and caregivers were possible anytime. During a 1-year period, the number of exacerbations did not differ between the telemonitored patients and the control group, but the number and duration of hospitalizations were significantly lower in the telemonitored group. Telemonitoring of the ventilator combined with teleconsultation was also used in children ventilated at home during the COVID-19 pandemic in order to reduce in-person clinic visits.[3] Most of the problems detected were able to be solved remotely.

A study investigating the experiences of patients, carers, and homecare professionals with telemonitoring in the management of NIV at home[48] found telemonitoring acceptable and considered it a useful addition to care. The risk of complacency associated with telemonitoring was raised in this study and requires further research. In a pediatric population, caregivers and parents indicated high satisfaction and no additional burden with the use of telemonitoring.[7,49]

Telemonitoring Non-Invasive Ventilation to Detect Exacerbations

Another potential clinical benefit of telemonitoring is the early detection of exacerbations, enabling necessary support to be provided remotely, and hospitalization to be prevented. A prospective controlled trial including 40 patients established on NIV for ALS compared conventional follow-up with office visits to follow-up based on telemonitoring of NIV.[50] Telemonitored data were reviewed weekly by the homecare provider and on request by the patient. Office visits, hospitalization, or a remote change of ventilator settings could be organized when necessary. During an average 1-year period, the number of office visits, emergency room visits, and hospitalizations were significantly lower in the telemonitored NIV group. Moreover, survival with NIV was much longer in the group of telemonitored NIV patients, although the results did not reach statistical significance. A cost analysis of telemonitoring NIV in ALS patients reported significant savings for the national health system when compared to conventional follow-up.[51]

Three studies have tried to determine whether daily monitoring of ventilator variables could help the early detection of exacerbations in COPD patients using NIV at home.[12–14] A change in RR is associated with the onset of an acute exacerbation in COPD. However, daily monitoring of RR was shown to have a low specificity for identifying exacerbations and is therefore unlikely to readily useful in clinical practice. In fact, false alerts may contribute to increased costs and worse outcomes. Artificial intelligence may prove to be helpful in defining individual, appropriate alerts using multiple variables.[52] In the meantime, an increase in RR, variation in daily usage, leaks, or a significant change in VT on 2 consecutive days should prompt the telemonitoring team to contact the patient and check their clinical condition.

SUMMARY

Telemonitoring of ventilators used at home for patients with chronic respiratory failure is a modern approach to medical practice, which is attractive to clinicians and well-accepted by patients and caregivers. Technical solutions for data transmission and platforms are rapidly improving. More precise data, the integration of physiologic measurements and the use of artificial intelligence to transform data into information are anticipated in the future. Telemonitoring is efficient, provided there is good coordination between the telemonitoring team, the homecare provider, the physician, and the patient. Remote adjustment of ventilator settings combined with educational support increases the value and effectiveness of telemonitoring. Telemonitoring can be used during the initiation of CPAP/NIV, in long-term stabilized patients, and for detecting clinical deterioration, with the aim of lessening the need for clinic visits and hospitalization. Clinical studies are required to determine the most

valuable variables to monitor, appropriate thresholds for alerts and the optimal coordination between stakeholders. An analysis of cost and clinical benefits for each subgroup of patients is also required. There is still a long journey ahead before telemonitoring becomes fully integrated into standard care.

CLINICS CARE POINTS

- Telemonitoring of CPAP/NIV allows rapid access and review of data that can optimize the efficiency of CPAP/NIV.
- Good coordination within the telemonitoring team is of critical importance.
- The patient is the major stakeholder in the telemonitoring process.
- Currently, telemonitoring still requires the attendance of the homecare provider in the home.
- Optimal settings and individualization of alerts is the key to efficient telemonitoring of CPAP/NIV.
- Remote adjustment of ventilator settings is complementary to telemonitoring.
- Telemonitoring CPAP/NIV may increase the quality of treatment delivery and reduce the need for hospitalizations.

DISCLOSURES

J.-M. Arnal is a consultant for Breas Medical and ResMed.

ACKNOWLEDGMENTS

Irène Vanicat and Nathalie Lemaire (ResMed France), Vivian Ducrot (ASV Santé), Myriam Benbassat Hoze, Sophie Charpin and Karine Dupré (Philips Respironics), Eric Royer (L3 Medical & Breas Medical), Antoine Delprat (Air Liquide), Alexandre Delcamp and Mélanie Eintrazi (Löwenstein). Caroline Brown for the English revision.

REFERENCES

1. Borel J-C, Palot A, Patout M. Technological advances in home non-invasive ventilation monitoring: reliability of data and effect on patient outcomes. Respirology 2019;24(12):1143–51.
2. Khirani S, Amaddeo A, Griffon L, et al. Follow-up and monitoring of children needing long term home ventilation. Front Pediatr 2020;8:330.

3. Onofri A, Pavone M, De Santis S, et al. Telemedicine in children with medical complexity on home ventilation during the COVID-19 pandemic. Pediatr Pulmonol 2021;56(6):1395–400.

4. Verbraecken J. Telemedicine in sleep-disordered breathing: expanding the horizons. Sleep Med Clin 2021;16(3):417–45.

5. Ackrivo J, Elman L, Hansen-Flaschen J. Telemonitoring for home-assisted ventilation: a narrative review. Ann Am Thorac Soc 2021;18(11):1761–72.

6. Duiverman M. "Tricks and tips for home mechanical ventilation" Home mechanical ventilation: set-up and monitoring protocols. Pulmonology 2021;27(2):144–50.

7. Trucco F, Pedemonte M, Racca F, et al. Tele-monitoring in paediatric and young home-ventilated neuromuscular patients: a multicentre case-control trial. J Telemed Telecare 2019;25(7):414–24.

8. Cantero C, Adler D, Pasquina P, et al. Long-term noninvasive ventilation in the geneva lake area: indications, prevalence, and modalities. Chest 2020;158(1):279–91.

9. Patout M, Lhuillier E, Kaltsakas G, et al. Long-term survival following initiation of home non-invasive ventilation: a European study. Thorax 2020;75(11):965–73.

10. Jolly G, Razakamanantsoa L, Fresnel E, et al. Defining successful non-invasive ventilation initiation: data from a real-life cohort. Respirology 2021;26(11):1067–75.

11. Boniol M, Kunjumen T, Nair TS, et al. The global health workforce stock and distribution in 2020 and 2030: a threat to equity and 'universal' health coverage? BMJ Glob Health 2022;7(6):e009316.

12. Blouet S, Sutter J, Fresnel E, et al. Prediction of severe acute exacerbation using changes in breathing pattern of COPD patients on home noninvasive ventilation. Int J Chronic Obstr Pulm Dis 2018;13:2577–86.

13. Borel J-C, Pelletier J, Taleux N, et al. Parameters recorded by software of non-invasive ventilators predict COPD exacerbation: a proof-of-concept study. Thorax 2015;70(3):284–5.

14. Jiang W, Chao Y, Wang X, et al. Day-to-day variability of parameters recorded by home noninvasive positive pressure ventilation for detection of severe acute exacerbations in COPD. Int J Chronic Obstr Pulm Dis 2021;16:727–37.

15. Arnal J-M, Oranger M, Gonzalez-Bermejo J. Monitoring systems in home ventilation. J Clin Med 2023;12(6):2163.

16. Contal O, Vignaux L, Combescure C, et al. Monitoring of noninvasive ventilation by built-in software of home bilevel ventilators: a bench study. Chest 2012;141(2):469–76.

17. Georges M, Adler D, Contal O, et al. Reliability of apnea-hypopnea index measured by a home Bi-level pressure support ventilator versus a polysomnographic assessment. Respir Care 2015;60(7):1051–6.

18. Fernandez Alvarez R, Rabec C, Rubinos Cuadrado G, et al. Monitoring noninvasive ventilation in patients with obesity hypoventilation syndrome: comparison between ventilator built-in software and respiratory polygraphy. Respiration 2017;93(3):162–9.

19. Zhu K, Rabec C, Gonzalez-Bermejo J, et al. Combined effects of leaks, respiratory system properties and upper airway patency on the performance of home ventilators: a bench study. BMC Pulm Med 2017;17(1):145.

20. Fresnel E, Vedrenne-Cloquet M, Lebret M, et al. Detection of simulated pediatric breathing by CPAP/noninvasive ventilation devices. Respir Care 2023;68(8):1087–96.

21. Khirani S, Delord V, Olmo Arroyo J, et al. Can the analysis of built-in software of CPAP devices replace polygraphy in children? Sleep Med 2017;37:46–53.

22. Sutter J, Cuvelier A, Lukaszewicz R, et al. Poor sleep quality and nocturnal home noninvasive ventilation: prevalence, risk factors and impact. Pulmonology 2023;18. S2531-S0437(23)00079-X.

23. Lebret M, Fresnel E, Prouvez N, et al. Responses of bilevel ventilators to unintentional leak: a bench study. Healthcare (Basel) 2022;10(12):2416.

24. Delorme M, Leroux K, Leotard A, et al. Noninvasive ventilation automated technologies: a bench evaluation of device responses to sleep-related respiratory events. Respir Care 2023;68(1):18–30.

25. Chen C, Wang J, Pang L, et al. Telemonitor care helps CPAP compliance in patients with obstructive sleep apnea: a systemic review and meta-analysis of randomized controlled trials. Ther Adv Chronic Dis 2020;11. 2040622320901625.

26. Bhattacharjee R, Benjafield AV, Armitstead J, et al. Adherence in children using positive airway pressure therapy: a big-data analysis. Lancet Digit Health 2020;2(2):e94–101.

27. Thomas A, Langley R, Pabary R. Feasibility and efficacy of active remote monitoring of home ventilation in pediatrics. Pediatr Pulmonol 2021;56(12):3975–82.

28. Palot A, Jaffuel D, Gouitaa M, et al. A place for apnea hypopnea index telemonitoring in preventing heart failure exacerbation? Sleep Med 2017;29:18–9.

29. Janssens J-P, Cantero C, Pasquina P, et al. Monitoring long term noninvasive ventilation: benefits, caveats and perspectives. Front Med 2022;9:874523.

30. Janssens JP, Borel JC, Pépin JL, et al. Nocturnal monitoring of home non-invasive ventilation: the contribution of simple tools such as pulse oximetry, capnography, built-in ventilator software and autonomic markers of sleep fragmentation. Thorax 2011;66(5):438–45.

31. Fauroux B, Khirani S, Amaddeo A, et al. Paediatric long term continuous positive airway pressure and

noninvasive ventilation in France: a cross-sectional study. Respir Med 2021;181:106388.

32. Jeganathan V, Rautela L, Conti S, et al. Typical within and between person variability in non-invasive ventilator derived variables among clinically stable, long-term users. BMJ Open Respir Res 2021;8(1): e000824.

33. Borel J-C, Bughin F, Texereau J. La télésurveillance du patient insuffisant respiratoire chronique en France : l'opportunité d'organiser une prise en charge efficiente [Telemonitoring of patients with chronic respiratory failure in France]. Rev Mal Respir 2023;9. S0761-8425(23)00172-9.

34. Drager LF, Malhotra A, Yan Y, et al. Adherence with positive airway pressure therapy for obstructive sleep apnea in developing vs. developed countries: a big data study. J Clin Sleep Med 2021;17(4): 703–9.

35. Hwang D, Chang JW, Benjafield AV, et al. Effect of telemedicine education and telemonitoring on continuous positive airway pressure adherence. The Tele-OSA Randomized Trial. Am J Respir Crit Care Med 2018;197(1):117–26.

36. Malhotra A, Crocker ME, Willes L, et al. Patient engagement using new technology to improve adherence to positive airway pressure therapy: a retrospective analysis. Chest 2018;153(4):843–50.

37. Dupuis-Lozeron E, Gex G, Pasquina P, et al. Development and validation of a simple tool for the assessment of home noninvasive ventilation: the S3-NIV questionnaire. Eur Respir J 2018;52(5): 1801182.

38. Soyez F, Ninot G, Herkert A, et al. Validation d'un questionnaire d'évaluation de l'exacerbation dans la BPCO : l'Exascore [Validation of an evaluation questionnaire for COPD acute exacerbations (Exascore)]. Rev Mal Respir 2016;33(1):17–24.

39. Windisch W, Freidel K, Schucher B, et al. The Severe Respiratory Insufficiency (SRI) Questionnaire: a specific measure of health-related quality of life in patients receiving home mechanical ventilation. J Clin Epidemiol 2003;56(8):752–9.

40. Petitjean T, Philit F, Germain-Pastenne M, et al. Sleep and respiratory function after withdrawal of noninvasive ventilation in patients with chronic respiratory failure. Respir Care 2008;53(10):1316–23.

41. Kampelmacher MJ. Moving from inpatient to outpatient or home initiation of non-invasive home mechanical ventilation. J Clin Med 2023;12(8):2981.

42. Réginault T, Bouteleux B, Wibart P, et al. At-home noninvasive ventilation initiation with telemonitoring in amyotrophic lateral sclerosis patients: a

retrospective study. ERJ Open Res 2023;9(1): 00438–2022.

43. Hazenberg A, Kerstjens HA, Prins SC, et al. Initiation of home mechanical ventilation at home: a randomised controlled trial of efficacy, feasibility and costs. Respir Med 2014;108(9):1387–95.

44. van den Biggelaar RJM, Hazenberg A, Cobben NAM, et al. A randomized trial of initiation of chronic noninvasive mechanical ventilation at home vs in-hospital in patients with neuromuscular disease and thoracic cage disorder: the Dutch homerun trial. Chest 2020;158(6):2493–501.

45. Duiverman ML, Vonk JM, Bladder G, et al. Home initiation of chronic non-invasive ventilation in COPD patients with chronic hypercapnic respiratory failure: a randomised controlled trial. Thorax 2020; 75(3):244–52.

46. Murphy PB, Patout M, Arbane G, et al. Cost-effectiveness of outpatient versus inpatient non-invasive ventilation setup in obesity hypoventilation syndrome: the OPIP trial. Thorax 2023;78(1):24–31.

47. Pontier-Marchandise S, Texereau J, Prigent A, et al. Home NIV treatment quality in patients with chronic respiratory failure having participated to the French nationwide telemonitoring experimental program (The TELVENT study). Respir Med Res 2023;84: 101028.

48. Mansell SK, Kilbride C, Wood MJ, et al. Experiences and views of patients, carers and healthcare professionals on using modems in domiciliary non-invasive ventilation (NIV): a qualitative study. BMJ Open Respir Res 2020;7(1):e000510.

49. Zhou J, Liu DB, Zhong JW, et al. Feasibility of a remote monitoring system for home-based non-invasive positive pressure ventilation of children and infants. Int J Pediatr Otorhinolaryngol 2012;76(12): 1737–40.

50. Pinto A, Almeida JP, Pinto S, et al. Home telemonitoring of non-invasive ventilation decreases healthcare utilisation in a prospective controlled trial of patients with amyotrophic lateral sclerosis. J Neurol Neurosurg Psychiatry 2010;81(11):1238–42.

51. Lopes de Almeida JP, Pinto A, Pinto S, et al. Economic cost of home-telemonitoring care for BiPAP-assisted ALS individuals. Amyotroph Lateral Scler 2012;13(6):533–7.

52. Orchard P, Agakova A, Pinnock H, et al. Improving prediction of risk of hospital admission in chronic obstructive pulmonary disease: application of machine learning to telemonitoring data. J Med Internet Res 2018;20(9):e263.

The Role of High Flow Nasal Therapy in Chronic Respiratory Failure

Emma Gray, FRACP, MPH[a,b,*], Collette Menadue, BAppSc(Phty), PhD[a]

KEYWORDS

- High-flow nasal therapy • Chronic hypercapnic respiratory failure • Hypercapnia
- Chronic obstructive pulmonary disease • Non-invasive ventilation

KEY POINTS

- High-flow nasal therapy (HFNT) leaves a constant reservoir of fresh gas in the conducting airways in patients with chronic hypercapnic respiratory failure (CHRF), resulting in reduced dead-space ventilation and subsequent reduction in work of breathing and arterial carbon dioxide.
- HFNT is easy to use, more tolerable, and associated with less pressure areas than non-invasive ventilation.
- Home HFNT and long-term oxygen therapy (LTOT) reduce exacerbations compared with LTOT alone in patients with chronic obstructive pulmonary disease and CHRF.

INTRODUCTION

Chronic hypercapnic respiratory failure (CHRF) occurs when there is an imbalance between the capacity of the respiratory pump and the load placed upon it, resulting in reduced alveolar ventilation (V_A) relative to carbon dioxide (CO_2) production. Untreated CHRF is associated with increased hospital admissions and health care costs, and decreased health-related quality of life (HRQL) and survival. Disease groups commonly presenting with CHRF include chronic obstructive pulmonary disease (COPD), obesity, and neuromuscular disease (NMD). Non-invasive ventilation (NIV) is a first line therapy for sleep-related hypoventilation and CHRF secondary to a range of etiologies.[1] Once established on long-term NIV, survival varies depending on diagnostic group with median survival of greater than 7 years reported in individuals with obesity hypoventilation syndrome with or without obstructive sleep apnoea (OSA) and in slowly progressive NMD.[2] Despite median survival

being lower at 1.1 years in rapidly progressive NMD and 2.7 years in COPD compared to other diagnostic groups, randomised controlled trials (RCTs) have shown a survival and HRQL benefit with long-term NIV compared to no NIV in both motor neuron disease (MND) and stable hypercapnic COPD.[3,4] NIV also prolonged the time to hospital readmission in severe COPD with persistent hypercapnia.[5] However, NIV is not tolerated by all patients with CHRF with intolerance rates of 20% to 25% being reported in people with COPD,[4,6,7] and in MND.[8] Furthermore, NIV may not be effective or feasible for some individuals. Consequently, alternative methods of respiratory support for nocturnal hypoventilation and CHRF are needed to optimise patient outcomes.

HFNT has been proposed as a strategy to provide respiratory support to individuals with CHRF, in particular in those with COPD. In the acute care setting, HFNT is widely used,[9] and guidelines recommend HFNT over conventional oxygen therapy (COT) and NIV for the

[a] Department of Respiratory and Sleep Medicine, Royal Prince Alfred Hospital, Camperdown, NSW, Australia;
[b] Central Clinical Medical School, The University of Sydney, Camperdown, NSW, Australia
* Corresponding author. Department of Respiratory and Sleep Medicine, Level 11, Royal Prince Alfred Hospital, Missenden Road Camperdown NSW 2050 Australia.
E-mail address: Emma.Gray@health.nsw.gov.au

Sleep Med Clin 19 (2024) 461–472
https://doi.org/10.1016/j.jsmc.2024.04.008
1556-407X/24/© 2024 Elsevier Inc. All rights reserved.

management of acute hypoxaemic respiratory failure, and HFNT over COT during breaks from NIV and in non-surgical patients at low risk of extubation failure.[10] Currently a trial of NIV remains first-line therapy in the management of acute hypercapnic respiratory failure secondary to an acute exacerbation of COPD (AECOPD), due to the lack of robust evidence demonstrating a reduction in mortality or intubation rates with HFNT.[10,11] However, if NIV is not tolerated, HFNT may be a reasonable alternative. Moving from the acute care setting to home, there is growing interest in the role of HFNT in the community. A recent survey with responses from approximately 25% of hospitals in the United Kingdom and Canada found that 10% of sites currently use HFNT in the community, despite the limited evidence-base.[9] To date, only one clinical practice guideline has recommended the use of HFNT in the home setting.[6]

The current review will focus on the role of home HFNT in people with CHRF, including the mechanisms of HFNT and how these may be beneficial in CHRF, short and long-term clinical effects of HFNT in CHRF, and discuss practical considerations and areas for future research for home HFNT.

PHYSIOLOGIC EFFECTS OF HIGH-FLOW NASAL THERAPY AND WHY HIGH-FLOW NASAL THERAPY MAY BE BENEFICIAL IN CHRONIC HYPERCAPNIC RESPIRATORY FAILURE

How Does High-Flow Nasal Therapy Work in Acute Hypoxaemic Respiratory Failure?

HFNT delivers heated and humidified air at high flow rates (up to 60L to 70L/min), with the fraction of inspired oxygen (Fio_2) adjustable (from 0.21 to 1.0) through changing the fraction of oxygen in the driving gas (**Fig. 1**). There are several proposed mechanisms contributing to the success of HFNT in acute hypoxaemic respiratory failure. High flow rates that match or exceed the patient's own inspiratory flow rate improve oxygenation by avoiding dilution with the entrainment of ambient air while minimising nasopharyngeal resistance, thereby decreasing the resistive work of breathing. This in turn decreases inspiratory effort and respiratory rate, and increases end-expiratory lung volume, alveolar recruitment, and homogeneous ventilation distribution.[12,13] In addition, the provision of warmed and humidified gas improves conductance and pulmonary compliance compared to dry, cooler gas,[14] as well as reducing the metabolic work associated with gas conditioning.[15]

Until recently, most studies examining the use of HFNT excluded patients with hypercapnia, likely because patients with CHRF are known to have a diminished respiratory drive when exposed to hyperoxia,[16] and HFNT was initially seen as an extension of COT. However, there is now increasing literature examining HFNT use in this patient population in both wakefulness and sleep.

Why High-Flow Nasal Therapy May be Advantageous in Chronic Hypercapnic Respiratory Failure

Nasopharyngeal dead-space washout

An increase in dead-space ventilation (V_D) through various mechanisms is one of the main and final common pathways leading to a reduction in V_A, and hence hypercapnia, in many types of CHRF (**Fig. 2**). In an animal model, Frizzola and colleagues first showed that the nasopharyngeal washout achieved by HFNT decreased arterial partial pressure of carbon dioxide ($Paco_2$) and increased arterial partial pressure of oxygen (Pao_2) in a flow-dependent manner until saturation was reached, independent of tracheal pressure generation alone.[17] This has subsequently been confirmed in human studies with the delivery of high flow rates to the nasopharynx. This provides a reservoir of well oxygenated gas proportional to flow rates, reducing V_D and thereby increasing V_A relative to minute ventilation (V_E), which in turn improves the efficacy of respiratory efforts.[18] This is a feature unique to open circuits as other modes of closed-circuit ventilation, such as NIV and mechanical ventilation, increase V_D.

Increased PEEP

HFNT has been shown to generate low levels (1 to 3cmH$_2$O) of positive pressure in healthy adults at flow rates in the range 20 to 60 L/min.[19] This has been confirmed in patients following elective cardiac surgery where positive pressures of 2cmH$_2$O were generated when the mouth was closed with HFNT delivered at 35 L/min.[20] Models have shown that an increased size of nasal cannula relative to the size of the nare, creating low leakage, as well as increasing flow rate can generate greater positive airway pressure.[21,22] In addition, PEEP has been shown to increase along with lung compliance,[23] while whether the mouth is open or closed also affects the pressure generated.[24] These increasing pressures inversely affect dead-space clearance by reducing the ability of expired air to escape.[20] It is unlikely that these subtle increases in pressure recruit previously closed alveoli, but rather may assist in keeping a proportion of small collapsing airways open.

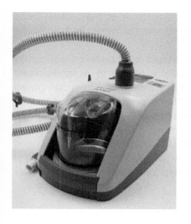 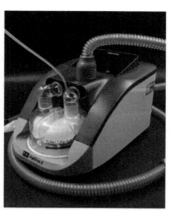

Fig. 1. High flow nasal therapy devices. (*A*) Airvo2 (Fisher & Paykel). (*B*) MyAirvo3 (Fisher & Paykel).

Airvo2 (Fisher & Paykel)   MyAirvo3 (Fisher & Paykel)

Improving V/Q mismatch

Retained secretions due to either atelectasis, ineffective cough, or mucous hypersecretion occurs in most causes of CHRF. This increases airway resistance, reduces lung compliance, and is associated with worsening V/Q mismatching and infection. The mucociliary epithelium responsible for clearance extends from the nasopharynx to the bronchioles and is highly sensitive to changes in temperature and humidity,[25] with airway resistance increasing in response to the inhalation of dry and cold gas, by reducing air flow in the upper conducting airways.[26,27] A small study of 10 bronchiectasis patients using HFNT for 3 hours a day, showed significantly improved mucociliary clearance (MCC) after 7 days of therapy.[28] Thus the provision of warmed and adequately humidified gas delivered at high flow has the physiologic effects of reducing airway constriction, enhancing mucociliary function, and facilitating clearance of secretions. This has the flow on effect of reducing atelectasis and improving V/Q matching. In addition, the metabolic load associated with gas conditioning is reduced if warmed, humidified gas is delivered to the conducting airways.[15]

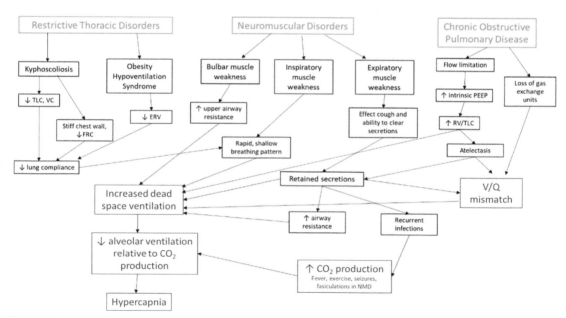

Fig. 2. Mechanisms through which respiratory disorders cause hypercapnia. CO_2, carbon dioxide; ERV, expiratory reserve volume; FRC, functional residual capacity; NMD, neuromuscular disorders; PEEP, positive end expiratory pressure; RV, residual volume; TLC, total lung capacity; V/Q, ventilation-perfusion; VC, vital capacity.

Interface tolerability

When considering long-term devices, the interface and mode of delivery is especially important for patient tolerability and comfort. Irrespective of the underlying pathology, the type of interface used in stable hypercapnic patients has a greater effect on NIV outcomes than the ventilatory mode that is used.[29] Pressure areas are of particular concern for closed circuit machines reliant on minimal leak, such as NIV, especially as time spent on the device increases, as significant tissue injury can lead to treatment breaks or discontinuation. Skin breakdown with HFNT is reported to be less, even after 24 hours of treatment, compared with NIV (3% vs 10%).[30]

Future directions: asymmetrical interface—the best of both worlds?

With current HFNT interfaces (**Fig. 3**A) the occurrence of PEEP and dead-space washout are inversely proportional. An interesting recent paper investigated the modeled effects of an asymmetrical nasal cannula interface (AI) (see **Fig. 3**B) compared with a symmetric interface (SI) had on PEEP and dead-space clearance.[31] This study confirmed that symmetric nares occlusion significantly worsens dead-space clearance, whereas asymmetrical nares occlusion increased dead-space clearance by nearly one-third. The AI significantly increased both PEEP and dead-space washout for every flow rate and respiratory rate trialed compared to the SI. Flow during inspiration was greatest through the larger prong, with the reverse true on expiration, creating reversal of flow between the nasal cavities and accelerating the unidirectional purging of expired air. The highest PEEP of 6.6cmH$_2$O was achieved with the larger AI at the highest flow rate of 60 L/min. Of note, the AI increased clearance three-fold at 20 L/min compared with SI even under COPD conditions of expiratory flow limitation and intrinsic PEEP. This higher efficiency of washout at lower flow rates is important, as it is these flow rates that are generally more tolerable in the home setting.[32]

The AI has been trialed in 10 patients with acute hypoxaemic respiratory failure in a randomised crossover trial at 40 L/min and 60 L/min compared with the SI.[33] The AI produced a significant reduction in minute ventilation of 13.5% at a flow rate of 40 L/min and 19.6% at a flow rate of 60 L/min compared with SI. This occurred without changes in gas exchange or pulmonary mechanics, suggesting the effect was due to upper airway clearance of CO$_2$.

SHORT TERM EFFECTS OF HIGH-FLOW NASAL THERAPY
Awake

Compared to spontaneous breathing

Over the short-term in healthy controls, HFNT has been shown to augment breathing patterns by reducing respiratory rate and increasing tidal volume (V_T), with resultant stable V_E during wakefulness.[34] In addition, HFNT significantly increases end-expiratory lung impedance, resulting in more uniform distribution of V_A between lung regions.[35] These changes are proportional to increasing flow rates.[36] An increase in end-expiratory lung impedance is associated with an increase in end-expiratory lung volume in intubated patients,[37] proposed to be important in alveolar recruitment.

Similar changes to breathing patterns are observed in patients with COPD, with decreases in respiratory rate, increases in V_T, and overall reductions in V_E following 8 hours of HFNT (20 L/min) resulting in improved V_A with reductions in Paco$_2$ (55.6 mm Hg to 50.5 mm Hg).[38] In the same study, Paco$_2$ remained constant and the V_T decreased in healthy volunteers.

Compared to conventional oxygen therapy

When compared to COT, 60-min of HFNT in stable COPD patients with both normocapnia and

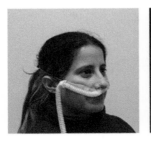

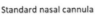

Standard nasal cannula

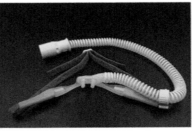

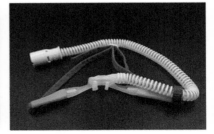

Asymmetrical nasal cannula

Fig. 3. Standard and asymmetrical nasal cannula. (*A*) Standard nasal cannula. (*B*) Asymmetrical nasal cannula (*Courtesy of* Elizabeth Lambrinos)

hypercapnia resulted in lower $Paco_2$ levels as well as lower Fio_2 requirements,[39] suggesting improvements to V_A with HFNT above COT.

Compared to non-invasive ventilation

Favourable changes in pulmonary mechanics and breathing patterns have also been shown in patients with stable hypercapnic COPD using HFNT over 30-min trials compared to NIV.[40] Both HFNT and NIV unloaded respiratory muscles through increased expiratory time and reduced respiratory rate, suggesting a change in the pressure-volume curve.[40]

HFNT also resulted in a flow-dependent reduction in $Paco_2$ following 2 hours of use among 54 hypercapnic COPD patients through a reduction in V_E via increased V_T and decreased respiratory rate accompanied by a minor flow dependent rise in mean airway pressure (1 to $3cmH_2O$).[41] In comparison, use of both nasal CPAP and NIV in this group led to increases in V_E. There were reductions in work of breathing with all modes of ventilatory support.

Although greater reductions in transcutaneous Pco_2 [mean difference -2.5 mm Hg (95% CI-4.5 to -0.5, $P = .016$)] occurred in a group of stable hypercapnic COPD patients with 60-min of NIV (IPAP $15cmH_2O$/EPAP $4cmH_2O$) compared with HFNT (45 L/min), HFNT was rated significantly easier to use and more comfortable than NIV.[42]

During Sleep

Compared to spontaneous breathing

During sleep in young healthy subjects, the application of HFNT up to 45 L/min resulted in stable oxygenation and respiratory rate despite a fall in V_E by about 20% as a result of a reduction in V_T.[34] Pinkham and colleagues confirmed that HFNT at 30 L/min in healthy adults reduced V_T by 20% in sleep, while maintaining gas exchange through the reduction of CO_2 rebreathing from the anatomic dead-space by 45%.[43]

In contrast to HFNT applied to COPD patients during wakefulness, where V_T has been shown to increase and respiratory rate decrease in proportion to flow rate,[41] during non-rapid eye movement (NREM) N2 sleep in COPD patients, HFNT (20 L/min) resulted in reduced V_E and V_T, without a change in Pco_2. This significant reduction in V_D was also seen during sleep in healthy controls. It has been shown that patients with a greater fraction of V_D at baseline, had the greatest reduction in V_D with HFNT.[44]

Compared to conventional oxygen therapy

In both healthy controls and stable COPD patients, HFNT (20 L/min) and COT (2 L/min) resulted in reduced V_E and V_T compared with spontaneous breathing in NREM (N2) sleep.[45] Interestingly, COT increased $Paco_2$ by approximately 3%, whereas HFNT reduced $Paco_2$ by around 4% and resulted in greater reductions in work of breathing measurements compared with COT. This is likely explained by a greater reduction in V_D and more effective V_A with HFNT compared with COT in COPD.

Special Populations

Obstructive sleep apnoea and high-flow nasal therapy

OSA is a common comorbidity in all of the conditions that predispose to CHRF. Although CPAP (median pressure $8cmH_2O$) has a more favourable effect on respiratory events and sleep efficiency compared to HFNT,[46] HFNT at median flow rates 60 L/min significantly improved apnoea-hypopnoea index (AHI) compared to baseline (median 10.8 events/hr vs 35.0 events/hr).[46] HFNT also significantly improved AHI in rapid eye movement (REM) sleep (10.2 vs 49.0), oxygen desaturation events (5.3 vs 29.4), and minimum oxygen saturation (88.5% vs 81%), but had no effect on sleep efficiency. In addition, a systematic review of COT compared with CPAP and HFNT showed COT and HFNT reduced AHI by one-third, compared with an 83% reduction with CPAP. There are no studies assessing carbon dioxide levels with HFNT, and no mention of the flow rates required.[47] Although HFNT is not as effective as positive airway pressure, it still provides beneficial alterations to sleep parameters compared to no therapy.

Neuromuscular patients and high-flow nasal therapy

In neuromuscular patients, multiple parameters of respiratory function are compromised (see **Fig. 1**). In a study of patients with chronic nocturnal hypoventilation already established on NIV, subjects were randomly assigned to 2-h treatment periods of either no treatment, NIV, or HFNT at 20 L/min or 50 L/min.[48] Gas exchange in N2 sleep was examined. The striking feature was that HFNT at 50 L/min was not tolerated in one-third of individuals, and one-quarter were unable to achieve 10 minutes of consecutive N2 sleep. Reasons were not elaborated. Only NIV resulted in a significant decrease of mean and maximum transcutaneous carbon dioxide ($TcCO_2$) when compared to no treatment. The authors concluded that HFNT was not a treatment alternative to NIV in non-dyspnoeic NMD patients. However, a case-series of 3 patients with MND, intolerant of NIV, showed immediate subjective improvements in dyspnea, secretion management and phonation, as well as 3-month improvement in daytime somnolence in 1 patient.[49] These benefits were achieved at modest flow rates of 20 to 30 L/min. More evidence is needed to establish safety; however, for these rapidly progressing neurodegenerative conditions where symptom management, not just gas exchange, is an important aspect of clinical care, HFNT may have a role.

MEDIUM TERM EFFECTS OF HIGH-FLOW NASAL THERAPY IN CHRONIC HYPERCAPNIC RESPIRATORY FAILURE
Compared to Long-Term Oxygen Therapy Alone

In a randomised crossover study in 29 participants with severe COPD and mild CHRF, 6 weeks of HFNT and LTOT improved HRQL, daytime $Paco_2$ and pH, and reduced nocturnal mean $TcCO_2$ compared to 6 weeks of LTOT alone.[50] Participants were advised to use HFNT (30 L/min) during sleep, and adherence was around 7 to 8 h/night. The magnitude of improvement in HRQL [mean change St George's Respiratory Questionnaire (SGRQ)−7.8 points] exceeded the reported minimal important difference of 4 points.[51] Similarly, the reduction in daytime and nocturnal Pco_2 of -4 mm Hg and -5 mm Hg respectively, may be clinically worthwhile and reflects an improvement in V_A, most likely achieved through anatomic deadspace washout during HFNT.

Compared to Non-Invasive Ventilation

In contrast to the comparison of HFNT with LTOT, no differences in HRQL or gas exchange were found when HFNT was compared to NIV in a randomised crossover study in 94 people with severe COPD and moderate-severe CHRF.[52] 6 weeks of HFNT and LTOT was compared with 6 weeks of NIV and LTOT. Participants were advised to use both therapies during sleep. Mean adherence was 5.2 h/night and 3.9 h/night respectively. Changes in Pco_2 and HRQL were not significantly different between HFNT and NIV. Of note, the mean reduction in Pco_2 was small, 3 mm Hg for HFNT and 4 mm Hg for NIV, particularly given the baseline Pco_2 of 57 ± 5 mm Hg. This likely reflects the low flow rate of 20 L/min used during HFNT, which may have limited dead-space washout. Slightly lower levels of pressure support were also used during NIV compared to current practice guidelines in COPD and therapy adherence was below that recommended for benefit.[45] Despite this, clinically worthwhile changes in HRQL were observed with both HFNT and NIV. Further studies are required to compare HFNT

and NIV when both modalities are set to optimally reduce Pco_2.

LONG TERM EFFECTS OF HIGH-FLOW NASAL THERAPY IN CHRONIC HYPERCAPNIC RESPIRATORY FAILURE
Compared to Long-Term Oxygen Therapy Alone

Two multicentre RCTs assessed the effects of home HFNT and LTOT compared to LTOT alone over 12 months in people with severe COPD and CHRF.[53,54] In the study by Storgaard and colleagues,[53] 52% of participants in the HFNT group and 60% in the control group were hypercapnic. In contrast, Nagata and coworkers[54] specifically recruited individuals with $Paco_2$ $\geq$45 mm Hg. Despite this, baseline $Paco_2$ was similar between studies (49 mm Hg vs 51 mm Hg respectively). Mean flow rates and adherence to HFNT were higher in the study by Nagata[54] (29 L/min vs 20 L/min, 7.3 h/day vs 6 h/day respectively). Over the 12-month period, 17/100 participants in the Storgaard study[53] were non-adherent to HFNT.

Both Storgaard[53] and Nagata[51] found a significant reduction in COPD exacerbation rates with HFNT compared with LTOT alone (3.1 exacerbations/patient/year vs 4.9, P<.001 and 1 exacerbation/patient/year vs 2.5, P = .002 respectively). Nagata[51] also reported a longer time to first exacerbation with HFNT. These findings are most likely mediated by an improvement in MCC due to humidification. In the Storgaard study,[53] HRQL remained stable in the HFNT group, while a clinically significant deterioration (4.4 points SGRQ total score) occurred in the LTOT group at 12 months. In contrast, a between group improvement in HRQL (4 point reduction SGRQ total score) was seen with HFNT in the Nagata study,[51] but only at week 24. Storgaard and colleagues[53] reported a significant improvement in $Paco_2$ at 12 months in favor of HFNT. However, the mean change was small (-2 mm Hg from baseline $Paco_2$) and influenced by a small rise in $Paco_2$ in the LTOT group. There were no between group differences in $Paco_2$ at 12 months in the Nagata study.[51] In addition, no significant between group differences were found in hospital admission rates, mortality, or sleep quality.

The long-term effects of home HFNT in COPD with CHRF have also been assessed in several systematic reviews and meta-analyses. Pitre[55] included data from Nagata,[50,54] Rea,[56] and Storgaard.[53] Rea[56] included a mixed group with COPD or bronchiectasis and it was unclear if participants had CHRF. The main findings from Pitre[55] were that home HFNT probably reduces exacerbations (RR 0.77 [95% CI 0.66–0.89]; moderate certainty), may reduce hospital admissions (RR 0.87 [95% CI 0.69–1.09]; low certainty), and may improve HRQL (mean difference (MD) −8.12 points SGRQ [95% CI -13.3 to −2.95]; low certainty). There was no effect on mortality. Another review by Zhang[57] included data from Nagata[50,54] and Storgaard,[58] the latter being a post-hoc analysis of an earlier Storgaard study[53] examining outcomes in hypercapnic participants. The main findings were that home HFNT may reduce COPD exacerbation rates (meta-analysis not performed), but does not improve $PaCO_2$ (mean difference −1.2 mm Hg, 95% CI -3.8–1.4) or PaO_2 (mean difference 2.8 mm Hg, 95% CI -1.4–7.0) compared to the control intervention. As participants included in these trials generally had mild CHRF, the findings may not be generalisable to individuals with more severe hypercapnia. A summary of medium and long-term HFNT randomised trials in COPD with CHRF is presented in **Table 1**.

DISCUSSION

NIV remains the first line therapy for sleep-related hypoventilation and CHRF for a range of conditions. In addition to the selection of appropriate settings and interface to optimally manage sleep-related hypoventilation and CHRF, adequate adherence is imperative to derive benefits such as improved survival.[2] Despite the potential benefits associated with NIV, a significant proportion of patients do not tolerate therapy. Remaining options are often limited to LTOT if hypoxaemic respiratory failure is present and/or palliative care for pharmacologic management of symptoms. However, due to the variety of physiologic effects associated with HFNT, including a reduction in V_D, generation of low levels of PEEP, enhanced mucociliary clearance (MCC), and a subsequent reduction in work of breathing, along with good tolerability and ease of use,[42] it is likely that HFNT will have a place in the management of CHRF in select individuals, particularly when NIV cannot be used.

The current evidence supporting long-term home HFNT is limited, and studies have primarily included individuals with severe COPD and hypoxaemic respiratory failure, with or without mild to moderate CHRF. In these groups, HFNT has consistently been shown to reduce the exacerbation rate,[53,54,56] most likely achieved via improved MCC secondary to humidification. Mucous plugs are common in COPD and were observed on chest CT scans in 22% of over 4000 individuals with COPD.[59] Of concern, the presence of mucous plugs in 1 to 2 medium-large size airways was associated with higher all-cause mortality (HR 1.15, 95% CI 1.02–1.29).[59] Reducing AECOPD is important both to patients, to improve HRQOL and survival, and the health system, to reduce hospital admissions and subsequent costs. The Danish Respiratory Society guideline currently recommends home HFNT for COPD with ≥2 severe AECOPD/year and persistent hypoxic respiratory failure, and consideration of home HFNT in severe bronchiectasis ± persistent hypoxaemic respiratory failure with frequent exacerbations.[6] In a post hoc analysis,[60] the effect of HFNT on exacerbations was shown to primarily occur in individuals with previous exacerbations, highlighting a sub-group to target in future research. The feasibility of using home HFNT may be limited, particularly if government funding or reimbursement for the HFNT device is not available. However, cost benefit analyses based on data from Storgaard and colleagues[53] have shown that home HFNT for COPD patients with chronic respiratory failure is very likely to be cost effective in both European and New Zealand health systems,[61,62] which may influence funding bodies as the evidence-base grows. Moving HFNT from hospital to the home also requires consideration of the cost and frequency of replacing of consumables, from both financial and sustainability perspectives.

The Danish Respiratory Society also recommends home HFNT in COPD with persistent hypercapnia where long-term NIV is recommended but not tolerated.[6] In COPD with CHRF, studies using NIV with high inspiratory pressures with or without high back-up rates to target a significant reduction in daytime $PaCO_2$ have shown benefits to survival,[4] and time to readmission.[5] Currently, home HFNT does not appear to reduce daytime $PaCO_2$ compared to LTOT alone in people with COPD and CHRF[54] and this may relate to the use of insufficient flow rates for adequate deadspace washout. The measurement of $PaCO_2$ in these long-term studies occurs during the day after the patient has been off HFNT for some time, in contrast to the short-term physiologic studies which measure $PaCO_2$ with HFNT in-situ. Consequently, if home HFNT is to be used during sleep, and if reducing sleep-related hypoventilation and daytime hypercapnia is the target, investigation into the optimal approach to titrate flow rates is required, and may require in-lab polysomnography with $TcCO_2$ monitoring to observe the effects of various flow rates on gas exchange during different sleep stages, particularly REM sleep. Despite recommending home HFNT to be used during sleep, none of the medium-long term studies discussed in this review performed

Table 1
Home high flow nasal therapy in stable COPD with chronic hypercapnic respiratory failure: Summary of randomised controlled trials

	Nagata and colleagues,[50] 2018, Ann Am Thorac Soc	Storgaard and colleagues,[53] 2018, Int J COPD	Braunlich and colleagues,[52] 2019, Int J COPD	Nagata and colleagues,[54] 2022, Am J Respir Crit Care Med
Population	n = 32 (29 analyzed), stable severe COPD with mild CHRF, $Paco_2$: Gp A 52(8) mm Hg; Gp B 52(7) mm Hg	n = 200 (200 analyzed), stable severe COPD with chronic hypoxic respiratory failure ± CHRF, $Paco_2$: HFNT group 49(10) mm Hg, LTOT group 48(8) mm Hg	n = 102 (94 analyzed), stable severe COPD with CHRF, $Paco_2$: 57(5) mm Hg	n = 104 (99 analyzed), stable COPD (GOLD stage 2–4) on LTOT with CHRF, $Paco_2$: HFNT group 51(5) mm Hg, LTOT group 51(5) mm Hg
Study design	Randomised crossover study 6/52 of each therapy	Parallel group multicentre RCT 12-mo follow-up	Randomised crossover study 6/52 of each therapy	Parallel group multicentre RCT 12-mo follow-up
Intervention	*Nocturnal HFNT + LTOT* Temperature: not reported Flow rate: Gp A 29(2)L/min; Gp B 30(5)L/min Supp O_2: same flow as LTOT HFNT adherence: Group A 7.1(1.5) h/day, Group B 8.6(2.9)h/day	*Nocturnal HFNT + LTOT* Temperature: not reported Flowrate 20 L/min Supp O_2: 1.6 L/min HFNT adherence: 6 h/day	*Nocturnal HFNT + LTOT* Temperature: 37°C Flow rate: 20(1)L/min Supp O_2: 2.2(0.9)L/min HFNT adherence: 5.2(3.3)h/day	*Nocturnal HFNT + LTOT* Temperature: aimed 37°C Flow rate: 29(5)L/min Supp O_2: 1.5(1)L/min HFNT adherence: 7.3(3)h/day
Comparison	*LTOT alone* Supp O_2: Gp A 1.4(0.9)L/min; Gp B 1.4(1.0)L/min	*LTOT alone* Supp O_2: 1.7 L/min	*NIV + LTOT* IPAP: 20.5(3.6) cmH_2O EPAP 4.6(1.2) cmH_2O BUR: 13(4) bpm Supp O_2: 2.0(0.7)L/min NIV adherence: 3.9(2.5)h/day	*LTOT alone* Supp O_2: 1.6(1)L/min
Outcomes	*HFNT + LTOT vs LTOT:* ↑HRQL -7.8 points SGRQ (95% CI -11.9 to −3.7); ↓$Paco_2$ -4 mm Hg (−7 to −2); ↓median nocturnal $TcCO_2$ -5 mm Hg (−8 to −2); ↑pH 0.02 (0.01–0.02)	*HFNT + LTOT vs LTOT:* ↓ exacerbation rate (3.12 vs 4.95/patient/year), ↓ dyspnoea, ↑HRQL, ↓$Paco_2$, ↑ 6-min walk test. No significant difference in hospital admission rates or all-cause mortality	*HFNT + LTOT vs NIV + LTOT:* No significant difference in Pco_2, HRQL (SGRQ, SRI), No significant difference from baseline in Po_2, spirometry, six-minute walk distance	*HFNT + LTOT vs LTOT:* ↓ moderate-severe exacerbation rate (1.0 vs 2.5/patient/year), ↑ time to exacerbation, ↑ HRQL, ↑SpO_2, improved lung function

(continued on next page)

Table 1 *(continued)*				
	Nagata and colleagues,[50] 2018, Ann Am Thorac Soc	Storgaard and colleagues,[53] 2018, Int J COPD	Braunlich and colleagues,[52] 2019, Int J COPD	Nagata and colleagues,[54] 2022, Am J Respir Crit Care Med
	No significant difference in Pao_2, dyspnoea, spirometry, lung volumes, 6-min walk test, physical activity			
Adverse events due to HFNT (n)	Night sweating (4), nasal discharge (1), insomnia (1), skin rash (1)	Nil recorded	Insomnia (1), epistaxis/nasal irritation (1)	Nil recorded

Data presented as mean (standard deviation) unless otherwise indicated. Ann Am Thorac Soc: Annals of the American Thoracic Society; Int J COPD: International journal of Chronic Obstructive Pulmonary Disease; Am J Respir Crit Care Med: American Journal of Respiratory & Critical Care Medicine; COPD: chronic obstructive pulmonary disease; CHRF: chronic hypercapnic respiratory failure; $Paco_2$: partial pressure of arterial carbon dioxide; HFNT: high flow nasal therapy; LTOT: long term oxygen therapy; HRQL: health related quality of life; SGRQ: St George's Respiratory Questionnaire; $TcCO_2$: transcutaneous carbon dioxide; Pao_2: partial pressure of arterial oxygen; Supp O_2: supplemental oxygen; RCT: randomised controlled trial; NIV: non-invasive ventilation; IPAP: inspiratory airway pressure; EPAP: expiratory positive airway pressure; BUR: back-up rate; SRI: Severe Respiratory Insufficiency questionnaire; GOLD, Global Initiative for Chronic Obstructive Lung Disease.

overnight monitoring of gas exchange to assess treatment efficacy. Investigation into the role of the asymmetric interface fits into this discussion, as at least from modeled data, it appears that both increased PEEP and dead-space washout is achievable at lower, more tolerable flow rates. In addition, further information is required regarding the minimum level of adherence required to derive benefits from home HFNT, and the optimum time to use HFNT that is, during sleep, wakefulness, or both needs clarification and may depend on the goals of therapy. Newer generation HFNT devices allow data to be downloaded (**Fig. 4**) and have remote monitoring capabilities. These features will be useful clinically to interpret treatment response, for research, and

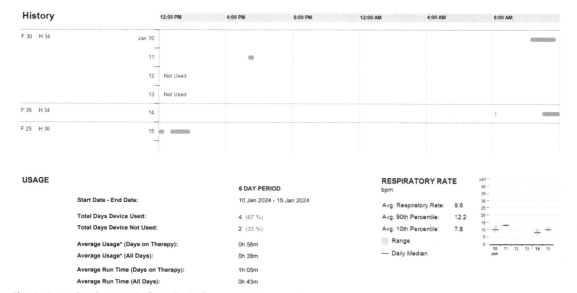

Fig. 4. Download example from high flow nasal therapy device

may be required by funding bodies to demonstrate adherence.

Another population that should theoretically benefit from domiciliary HFNT are people with NMD, especially MND, where symptom improvement is just as important as improvement in gas exchange. While only one study examining the effects of HFNT during N2 sleep in NMD patients already established on NIV has been performed,[48] low level evidence suggests that HFNT is tolerable and improves debilitating sleep-symptoms.[49] High-quality studies examining HFNT as a potential therapy where NIV is deemed intolerable or undesirable in these patients are warranted.

SUMMARY

Perhaps the greatest achievement of HFNT is that during spontaneous breathing without volume or pressure support, it works to reduce V_D and work of breathing, generating low levels of PEEP, and helping with secretion management via a tolerable and easy to use interface. Because of these favourable features, while HFNC is unlikely surpass NIV in the treatment of CHRF, there will likely be a place for this therapy, especially in those patients intolerant of NIV. The asymmetrical interface is of interest, given that it can provide increased dead-space washout more effectively at more tolerable lower flow rates.

CLINICS CARE POINTS

- Long term HFNT can reduce COPD exacerbation rates compared to LTOT alone in those with severe COPD and CHRF. This is most likely related to humidification and improved mucociliary clearance.
- HFNT may be an alternative to select patients with CHRF from other causes who are intolerant to NIV and would benefit from improved dead space washout and humidification.

DISCLOSURES

The authors have no conflicts of interest to declare relating to this review.

REFERENCES

1. Windisch W, Geiseler J, Simon K, et al. On behalf of the guideline C. German National guideline for treating chronic respiratory failure with invasive and non-invasive ventilation - Revised Edition 2017: Part 2. Respiration 2018;96(2):171–203.
2. Patout M, Lhuillier E, Kaltsakas G, et al. Long-term survival following initiation of home non-invasive ventilation: a European study. Thorax 2020;75(11):965–73.
3. Bourke SC, Tomlinson M, Williams TL, et al. Effects of non-invasive ventilation on survival and quality of life in patients with amyotrophic lateral sclerosis: a randomised controlled trial. Lancet Neurol 2006; 5(2):140–7.
4. Kohnlein T, Windisch W, Kohler D, et al. Non-invasive positive pressure ventilation for the treatment of severe stable chronic obstructive pulmonary disease: a prospective, multicentre, randomised, controlled clinical trial. Lancet Respir Med 2014;2(9):698–705.
5. Murphy PB, Rehal S, Arbane G, et al. Effect of home noninvasive ventilation with oxygen therapy vs oxygen therapy alone on hospital readmission or death after an acute COPD exacerbation: a randomized clinical trial. JAMA 2017;317(21):2177–86.
6. Weinreich UM, Juhl KS, Søby Christophersen M, et al. The Danish respiratory society guideline for long-term high flow nasal cannula treatment, with or without supplementary oxygen. European Clinical Respiratory Journal 2023;10(1):2178600.
7. Murphy P, Lyall R, Hart N, et al. Assessment of respiratory muscle strength in motor neurone disease: is asking enough? Eur Respir J 2010;35(2):245.
8. Bertella E, Banfi P, Paneroni M, et al. Early initiation of night-time NIV in an outpatient setting: a randomized non-inferiority study in ALS patients. Eur J Phys Rehabil Med 2017;53(6):892–9.
9. Alnajada A, Blackwood B, Messer B, et al. International survey of high-flow nasal therapy use for respiratory failure in adult patients. J Clin Med 2023; 12(12).
10. Oczkowski S, Ergan B, Bos L, et al. ERS clinical practice guidelines: high-flow nasal cannula in acute respiratory failure. Eur Respir J 2022;59(4).
11. Ovtcharenko N, Ho E, Alhazzani W, et al. High-flow nasal cannula versus non-invasive ventilation for acute hypercapnic respiratory failure in adults: a systematic review and meta-analysis of randomized trials. Crit Care 2022;26(1):348.
12. Mauri T, Turrini C, Eronia N, et al. Physiologic effects of high-flow nasal cannula in acute hypoxemic respiratory failure. Am J Respir Crit Care Med 2017; 195(9):1207–15.
13. Corley A, Caruana LR, Barnett AG, et al. Oxygen delivery through high-flow nasal cannulae increase end-expiratory lung volume and reduce respiratory rate in post-cardiac surgical patients. Br J Anaesth 2011;107(6):998–1004.
14. Greenspan JS, Wolfson MR, Shaffer TH. Airway responsiveness to low inspired gas temperature in preterm neonates. J Pediatr 1991;118(3):443–5.

15. Dysart K, Miller TL, Wolfson MR, et al. Research in high flow therapy: mechanisms of action. Respir Med 2009;103(10):1400–5.

16. Sassoon CS, Hassell KT, Mahutte CK. Hyperoxic-induced hypercapnia in stable chronic obstructive pulmonary disease. Am Rev Respir Dis 1987; 135(4):907–11.

17. Frizzola M, Miller TL, Rodriguez ME, et al. High-flow nasal cannula: impact on oxygenation and ventilation in an acute lung injury model. Pediatr Pulmonol 2011;46(1):67–74.

18. Wettstein R, Peters J, Shelledy D. Pharyngeal oxygen concentration in normal subjects wearing high flow nasal cannula. Respir Care 2004; 49(11):1444.

19. Groves N, Tobin A. High flow nasal oxygen generates positive airway pressure in adult volunteers. Aust Crit Care 2007;20(4):126–31.

20. Parke R, McGuinness S, Eccleston M. Nasal high-flow therapy delivers low level positive airway pressure. Br J Anaesth 2009;103(6):886–90.

21. Pinkham M, Tatkov S. Effect of flow and cannula size on generated pressure during nasal high flow. Crit Care 2020;24(1):248.

22. Pinkham MI, Domanski U, Franke KJ, et al. Effect of respiratory rate and size of cannula on pressure and dead-space clearance during nasal high flow in patients with COPD and acute respiratory failure. J Appl Physiol (1985) 2022;132(2):553–63.

23. Luo JC, Lu MS, Zhao ZH, et al. Positive end-expiratory pressure effect of 3 high-flow nasal cannula devices. Respir Care 2017;62(7):888–95.

24. Braunlich J, Mauersberger F, Wirtz H. Effectiveness of nasal highflow in hypercapnic COPD patients is flow and leakage dependent. BMC Pulm Med 2018;18(1):14.

25. Williams R, Rankin N, Smith T, et al. Relationship between the humidity and temperature of inspired gas and the function of the airway mucosa. Crit Care Med 1996;24(11):1920–9.

26. Fontanari P, Burnet H, Zattara-Hartmann MC, et al. Changes in airway resistance induced by nasal inhalation of cold dry, dry, or moist air in normal individuals. J Appl Physiol 1996;81(4):1739–43.

27. Fontanari P, Zattara-Hartmann MC, Burnet H, et al. Nasal eupnoeic inhalation of cold, dry air increases airway resistance in asthmatic patients. Eur Respir J 1997;10(10):2250–4.

28. Hasani A, Chapman TH, McCool D, et al. Domiciliary humidification improves lung mucociliary clearance in patients with bronchiectasis. Chron Respir Dis 2008;5(2):81–6.

29. Navalesi P, Fanfulla F, Frigerio P, et al. Physiologic evaluation of noninvasive mechanical ventilation delivered with three types of masks in patients with chronic hypercapnic respiratory failure. Crit Care Med 2000;28(6):1785–90.

30. Stephan F, Barrucand B, Petit P, et al. High-flow nasal oxygen vs noninvasive positive airway pressure in hypoxemic patients after cardiothoracic surgery: a randomized clinical trial. JAMA 2015; 313(23):2331–9.

31. Tatkov S, Rees M, Gulley A, et al. Asymmetrical nasal high flow ventilation improves clearance of CO_2 from the anatomical dead space and increases positive airway pressure. J Appl Physiol 2023;134(2):365–77.

32. Narang I, Carberry JC, Butler JE, et al. Physiological responses and perceived comfort to high-flow nasal cannula therapy in awake adults: effects of flow magnitude and temperature. J Appl Physiol 2021; 131(6):1772–82.

33. Slobod D, Spinelli E, Crotti S, et al. Effects of an asymmetrical high flow nasal cannula interface in hypoxemic patients. Crit Care 2023;27(1):145.

34. Mündel T, Feng S, Tatkov S, et al. Mechanisms of nasal high flow on ventilation during wakefulness and sleep. J Appl Physiol 2013;114(8): 1058–65.

35. Plotnikow GA, Thille AW, Vasquez DN, et al. Effects of high-flow nasal cannula on end-expiratory lung impedance in semi-seated healthy subjects. Respir Care 2018;63(8):1016–23.

36. Parke RL, Bloch A, McGuinness SP. Effect of very-high-flow nasal therapy on airway pressure and end-expiratory lung impedance in healthy volunteers. Respir Care 2015;60(10):1397–403.

37. Hinz J, Hahn G, Neumann P, et al. End-expiratory lung impedance change enables bedside monitoring of end-expiratory lung volume change. Intensive Care Med 2003;29(1):37–43.

38. Bräunlich J, Beyer D, Mai D, et al. Effects of nasal high flow on ventilation in volunteers, COPD and idiopathic pulmonary fibrosis patients. Respiration 2013;85(4):319–25.

39. Vogelsinger H, Halank M, Braun S, et al. Efficacy and safety of nasal high-flow oxygen in COPD patients. BMC Pulm Med 2017;17(1):143.

40. Pisani L, Fasano L, Corcione N, et al. Change in pulmonary mechanics and the effect on breathing pattern of high flow oxygen therapy in stable hypercapnic COPD. Thorax 2017;72(4):373–5.

41. Braunlich J, Kohler M, Wirtz H. Nasal highflow improves ventilation in patients with COPD. Int J Chronic Obstr Pulm Dis 2016;11:1077–85.

42. McKinstry S, Singer J, Baarsma JP, et al. Nasal high-flow therapy compared with non-invasive ventilation in COPD patients with chronic respiratory failure: a randomized controlled cross-over trial. Respirology 2019;24(11):1081–7.

43. Pinkham M, Burgess R, Mündel T, et al. Nasal high flow reduces minute ventilation during sleep through a decrease of carbon dioxide rebreathing. J Appl Physiol 2019;126(4):863–9.

44. Biselli P, Fricke K, Grote L, et al. Reductions in dead space ventilation with nasal high flow depend on physiologic dead space volume: metabolic hood measurements during sleep in patients with COPD and controls. Eur Respir J 2018;51: 1702251.

45. Biselli PJ, Kirkness JP, Grote L, et al. Nasal high-flow therapy reduces work of breathing compared with oxygen during sleep in COPD and smoking controls: a prospective observational study. J Appl Physiol 2017;122(1):82–8.

46. Yu C-C, Huang C-Y, Hua C-C, et al. High-flow nasal cannula compared with continuous positive airway pressure in the treatment of obstructive sleep apnea. Sleep Breath 2022;26(2):549–58.

47. Ruan B, Nagappa M, Rashid-Kolvear M, et al. The effectiveness of supplemental oxygen and high-flow nasal cannula therapy in patients with obstructive sleep apnea in different clinical settings: a systematic review and meta-analysis. J Clin Anesth 2023;88:111144.

48. Meyer AC, Spiesshoefer J, Siebers NC, et al. Effects of nasal high flow on nocturnal hypercapnia, sleep, and sympathovagal balance in patients with neuromuscular disorders. Sleep Breath 2021;25(3): 1441–51.

49. Anton AL, Shah J. Heated Humidified High Flow Nasal Cannula in ALS: Salvage Therapy for NPPV Intolerance. D41 Case reports in transplant and neuromuscular disease. A6750-A6750.

50. Nagata K, Kikuchi T, Horie T, et al. Domiciliary high-flow nasal cannula oxygen therapy for patients with stable hypercapnic chronic obstructive pulmonary disease. a multicenter randomized crossover trial. Ann Am Thorac Soc 2018;15(4):432–9.

51. Jones PW. St. George's respiratory questionnaire: MCID. COPD 2005;2(1):75–9.

52. Bräunlich J, Dellweg D, Bastian A, et al. Nasal high-flow versus noninvasive ventilation in patients with chronic hypercapnic COPD. Int J Chronic Obstr Pulm Dis 2019;14:1411–21.

53. Storgaard LH, Hockey HU, Laursen BS, et al. Long-term effects of oxygen-enriched high-flow nasal cannula treatment in COPD patients with chronic hypoxemic respiratory failure. Int J Chronic Obstr Pulm Dis 2018;13:1195–205.

54. Nagata K, Horie T, Chohnabayashi N, et al. Home high-flow nasal cannula oxygen therapy for stable hypercapnic COPD: a randomized clinical trial. Am J Respir Crit Care Med 2022;206(11):1326–35.

55. Pitre T, Abbasi S, Su J, et al. Home high flow nasal cannula for chronic hypercapnic respiratory failure in COPD: a systematic review and meta-analysis. Respir Med 2023;219:107420.

56. Rea H, McAuley S, Jayaram L, et al. The clinical utility of long-term humidification therapy in chronic airway disease. Respir Med 2010;104(4):525–33.

57. Zhang L, Wang Y, Ye Y, et al. Comparison of high-flow nasal cannula with conventional oxygen therapy in patients with hypercapnic chronic obstructive pulmonary disease: a systematic review and meta-analysis. Int J Chronic Obstr Pulm Dis 2023;18:895–906.

58. Storgaard LH, Hockey HU, Weinreich UM. Development in PaCO(2) over 12 months in patients with COPD with persistent hypercapnic respiratory failure treated with high-flow nasal cannula-post-hoc analysis from a randomised controlled trial. BMJ Open Respir Res 2020;7(1).

59. Diaz AA, Orejas JL, Grumley S, et al. Airway-occluding mucus plugs and mortality in patients with chronic obstructive pulmonary disease. JAMA 2023;329(21):1832–9.

60. Weinreich UM. Domiciliary high-flow treatment in patients with COPD and chronic hypoxic failure: in whom can we reduce exacerbations and hospitalizations? PLoS One 2019;14(12):e0227221.

61. Sørensen SS, Storgaard LH, Weinreich UM. Cost-effectiveness of domiciliary high flow nasal cannula treatment in COPD patients with chronic respiratory failure. Clinicoecon Outcomes Res 2021;13:553–64.

62. Milne RJ, Hockey HU, Garrett J. Hospital cost savings for sequential COPD patients receiving domiciliary nasal high flow therapy. Int J Chronic Obstr Pulm Dis 2022;17:1311–22.

Impact of Disease-modifying Therapies on Respiratory Function in People with Neuromuscular Disorders

Lena Xiao, MD, MSc[a,b], Reshma Amin, MD, MSc[c,d],*

KEYWORDS

- Neuromuscular disease • Spinal muscular atrophy • Duchenne muscular dystrophy • Nusinersen
- Risdiplam • Onasemnogene abeparvovec • Eteplirsen • Ataluren

KEY POINTS

- Disease-modifying therapies for SMA and DMD are rapidly shifting current paradigms of care.
- Disease-modifying therapies generally attenuate the natural trajectory of respiratory decline but do not reverse disease.
- Ongoing respiratory surveillance and monitoring are an integral component of care for people on disease-modifying therapies.

INTRODUCTION

Neuromuscular disorders (NMDs) are genetic disorders that affect muscular function. Progressive respiratory muscle weakness is a common complication in NMD. The use of respiratory therapies for cough augmentation, lung volume recruitment, and nocturnal respiratory support has helped to mitigate respiratory decline,[1,2] highlighting the importance of respiratory surveillance and therapies. Although clinical guidelines currently exist for the respiratory surveillance and management of people with NMDs, the paradigm of care is rapidly changing as novel disease-modifying therapies alter disease trajectories, outcomes, and expectations. It is therefore of paramount importance to understand how disease-modifying therapies alter the respiratory function. This article provides an overview on therapeutic advances for spinal muscular atrophy (SMA) and Duchenne muscular dystrophy (DMD) in the last 10 years, with a focus on respiratory outcomes.

SPINAL MUSCULAR ATROPHY

SMA is an autosomal recessive NMD due to the homozygous deletion or mutation in the *SMN1* gene.[3] This causes a lack of functional survival motor neuron (SMN) protein, which leads to the degeneration of anterior horn cells in the spinal cord and progressive muscular weakness. In the most severe form, SMA leads to death at a median of 8 to 13 months without supportive treatment.[4–6]

Pulmonary Function in Natural History Cohorts

Pulmonary function test data

Respiratory function in children with SMA is commonly monitored using pulmonary function

---

[a] Division of Respiratory Medicine, British Columbia Children's Hospital, 4480 Oak Street, Room 1C31A, Vancouver, British Columbia, V6H 3V4, Canada; [b] University of British Columbia, Vancouver, Canada; [c] Division of Respiratory Medicine, The Hospital for Sick Children, 175 Elizabeth Street, 16-14-026, Patient Support Center, Toronto, ON, M5G2G3, Canada; [d] University of Toronto, Toronto, Canada
* Corresponding author. The Hospital for Sick Children, 16-14-026, Patient Support Center, 175 Elizabeth Street, Toronto, Ontario, M5G 2G3, Canada.
E-mail address: reshma.amin@sickkids.ca

Sleep Med Clin 19 (2024) 473–483
https://doi.org/10.1016/j.jsmc.2024.04.004
1556-407X/24/© 2024 Elsevier Inc. All rights reserved.

tests (PFTs) because patients with abnormal pulmonary function are at higher risk of requiring noninvasive ventilation (NIV).[7] Treatment-naive patients with early-onset SMA (types 1c–3a) typically experience progressively declining lung function in childhood with relative stabilization during adulthood, whereas people with later onset SMA types 3b and 4 have normal lung function.[8] An 8 year retrospective observational study of 437 treatment-naive patients (SMA type 2 = 348, nonambulant SMA type 3 = 89) found that the percent predicted forced vital capacity (FVC) declined by 4.2%/year between 5 and 13 years followed by a slower decline of 1.0%/year in people with SMA type 2 and by 6.3%/year between 8 and 13 years followed by a slower decline of 0.9%/year in people with nonambulant SMA type 3.[9]

Polysomnogram data

Treatment-naïve children with SMA commonly have sleep-disordered breathing, with increased severity in more severe SMA phenotypes. In a cross-sectional study of treatment-naive children with SMA, those with SMA type 1 (n = 6) had a median (range) apnea–hypopnea index (AHI) of 12.3 (5.9–31.4) events/hour at a median (range) age of 1.0 (0.25–6.25) years.[10] Children with SMA type 2 (n = 16; polysomnographies [PSGs] at a median [range] age of 10.6 [2.8–18.8] years) and SMA type 3 (n = 9; PSGs at a median [range] age of 9.5 [3.2–15.4] years) had a median (range) AHI of 3.0 (0.7–44.0) events/hour and 2.1 (1.1–18.2) events/hour, respectively.[10]

There is evidence that presymptomatic infants with SMA types 1 to 2 may have subtle respiratory disease. In 8 infants diagnosed by newborn screening (6 treatment-naive and 2 received one dose of nusinersen), AHIs were elevated compared to external healthy infant data, with a median (interquartile range [IQR]) AHI, obstructive AHI, and central AHI of 26.1 (13.5–35.8), 4.1 (0.1–12.6), 19.3 (10.8–34.0) events/hour, respectively, at a median (IQR) age of 3.6 (2.9–7.0) weeks.[11]

DISEASE-MODIFYING THERAPIES FOR SPINAL MUSCULAR ATROPHY

There are 3 disease-modifying therapies that are currently approved by the US Food and Drug Administration (FDA) for the treatment of SMA (**Table 1**).

Nusinersen

Nusinersen is an intrathecally administered antisense oligonucleotide therapy that promotes production of functional SMN protein through the modification of SMN2 messenger ribonucleic acid (mRNA) splicing.[12]

Nusinersen for early-onset spinal muscular atrophy

The ENDEAR trial was a 6 month, double-blind, randomized controlled trial of nusinersen versus sham control in 121 symptomatic infants aged 7 months or younger (nusinersen = 80, sham control = 41).[13] Infants treated with nusinersen had improved motor function, increased survival, and delayed ventilation dependence.[13] The risk for the composite endpoint of death or the use of permanent-assisted ventilation, defined as ventilation for ≥16 hours/day continuously for greater than 21 days in the absence of an acute reversible event or tracheostomy, was 47% lower in the nusinersen group (hazard ratio, 0.53; 95% confidence interval [CI] 0.32–0.89; P = .005).[13] However, there was no difference in permanent ventilation dependence.[13]

The effect of nusinersen on presymptomatic infants treated at ≤6 weeks was evaluated in the phase 2, open-label, single-arm NURTURE trial (n = 25).[14,15] All 25 children (2 SMN2 copies = 15; 3 SMN2 copies = 10) were alive and free from permanent ventilation after 5 years of nusinersen treatment.[14] Of these children, 3 received NIV for 9 to 10 hours/day and one child used cough augmentation twice daily.[14] Many studies of nusinersen in children with early-onset SMA outside of clinical trial conditions suggest the need for stable or increased ventilatory support in the short and long term.[16–29]

Polysomnographic data are the primary type of objective respiratory data currently available for infants with SMA. Chacko and colleagues conducted a prospective observational cohort study in 28 children with SMA (aged 0.1–18.6 years, SMA type 1 = 7, SMA type 2 = 12, SMA type 3 = 9) during the first year of nusinersen therapy.[22] In children with SMA type 1 (median age 0.42 years at study initiation), the total AHI improved from a baseline median (IQR) of 4.4 (0.8–8.3) events/hour to 3.4 (1.3–6.3) events/hour after 1 year of nusinersen (P = .04).[22] In a separate observational study including a subset of 8 nusinersen-treated symptomatic children with SMA type 1 (all had 2 SMN2 copies), all children had sleep-disordered breathing despite treatment with nusinersen (median [IQR] AHI 9.5 [6.2–13.8] events/hour; median [IQR] age at the time of PSG was 9.4 [5.3–14.0] months).[21] The elevated AHI was primarily driven by central respiratory events (median [IQR] central AHI 4.1 [1.8–10.0] events/hour).[21]

Table 1
Disease-modifying therapies for spinal muscular atrophy and Duchenne muscular dystrophy

Treatment	Mechanism	Method of Administration	Commonly Published Respiratory Endpoints	Year of FDA Approval
Spinal muscular atrophy				
Nusinersen (Spinraza)	Antisense oligonucleotide splicing modifier of *SMN2*	Intrathecal injection	FVC, AHI	2016
Onasemnogene abeparvovec (Zolgensma)	Adeno-associated virus vector-based gene therapy	One time intravenous injection	FVC, AHI	2019
Risdiplam (Evrysdi)	Small molecule splicing modifier of *SMN2*	Once daily oral medication	FVC, MIP, MEP, PCF, SNIP	2020
Duchenne muscular dystrophy				
Ataluren (Translarna)	Small molecule resulting in read through of premature stop codons	Three times daily oral medication	FVC	Not approved by FDA; approved by EMA
Eteplirsen (Exondys 51)	Antisense oligonucleotide resulting in *DMD* exon 51 skipping	Once weekly intravenous infusion	FVC, MIP, MEP	2016
Golodirsen (Vyondys 53)	Antisense oligonucleotide resulting in *DMD* exon 53 skipping	Once weekly intravenous infusion	FVC	2019
Viltolarsen (Viltepso)	Antisense oligonucleotide resulting in *DMD* exon 53 skipping	Once weekly intravenous infusion	N/A	2020
Casimersen (Amondys 45)	Antisense oligonucleotide resulting in *DMD* exon 45 skipping	Once weekly intravenous infusion	N/A	2021
Delandistrogene moxeparvovec-rokl (Elevidys)	Adeno-associated virus vector-based gene therapy	One time intravenous injection	N/A	2023

Abbreviations: AHI, apnea–hypopnea index; EMA, European Medicines Agency; FDA, Food and Drug Administration; FVC, forced vital capacity; MEP, maximal expiratory pressure; MIP, maximal inspiratory pressure; PCF, peak cough flow; SNIP, sniff inspiratory pressure.

Nusinersen for later onset spinal muscular atrophy

The CHERISH trial was a double-blind, sham-controlled trial of nusinersen in 126 children with SMA types 2 and 3 aged 2 to 12 years (nusinersen = 84, control = 42).[30] A significant improvement in motor function favoring nusinersen after 15 months was reported, but respiratory outcomes were not assessed.[30]

The 2 part EMBRACE trial evaluated nusinersen therapy in children with early-onset or late-onset SMA who were ineligible for the ENDEAR and CHERISH trials.[31] The trial was comprised of 2 parts; participants were randomized to nusinersen (n = 14) or sham (n = 7) in part 1, and subsequently received open-label nusinersen for 24 months in part 2.[31] Motor milestone responder rates were highest in patients who received nusinersen throughout the study.[31] The mean percentage time on ventilator support was 11.3% in participants treated with nusinersen throughout the study compared to 29.8% in participants who received sham in part 1.[31] However, the results must be interpreted with caution because the treatment arms in part 1 were unbalanced; 3 of 14 (21%) participants randomized to nusinersen were on ventilation at baseline compared to 4 of 7 (57%) randomized to sham.[31]

Most data regarding respiratory outcomes after treatment with nusinersen in later onset SMA come from observational studies. Although Chacko and colleagues did not observe statistically significant AHI improvements for nusinersen-treated patients with SMA types 2 and 3,[22] they reported a significant improvement in the oxygen saturation nadir from 87.9% to 92.3% (mean difference 95% CI 1.24%–7.63%; $P = .01$) and total AHI from 13.96 to 2.9 events/hour (mean difference 95% CI −21.16 to −0.95 events/hour; $P = .03$) during the 2 year post-nusinersen therapy as compared to the 2 year pre-nusinersen therapy (SMA type 1 = 2, SMA type 2 = 10, SMA type 3 = 4; pre-nusinersen PSGs at mean age 7.5 years).[32]

Three small studies have reported PFT outcomes in children with SMA types 2 and 3 treated with nusinersen. Chacko and colleagues reported a decreased rate of decline of percent predicted FVC in children with SMA type 2 receiving nusinersen therapy from a mean of −5.86% (95% CI −7.60 to – 4.11) during the 2 years prior to nusinersen initiation compared with a mean of −1.03% (95% CI −3.55–1.50) during the first year of nusinersen therapy.[22] There was also a non-statistically significant trend toward a decreased rate of decline in children with SMA type 3.[22] The remaining 2 studies did not find a significant change in percent predicted FVC with nusinersen therapy.[32,33] Similarly, adults with SMA types 2 and 3 did not demonstrate improvement in the forced expiratory volume in 1 second (FEV1)[34] or FVC[35] following nusinersen initiation.

Onasemnogene Abeparvovec

Onasemnogene abeparvovec is an adeno-associated viral vector that encodes the SMN1 gene and is the first gene replacement therapy approved for SMA.

Onasemnogene abeparvovec for early-onset spinal muscular atrophy

The phase 1 START trial of 15 symptomatic infants with SMA type 1 less than 8 month old (high dose cohort = 12, low dose cohort = 3) demonstrated motor improvements in 11 of 12 study participants in the high dose cohort and survival of all children at 20 months of age without the need for permanent ventilatory assistance, which was considerably better than a survival rate of 8% in a natural history cohort.[36] Of the 12 infants who received high dose therapy, 5 infants required NIV by 24 month post-treatment, including 3 infants who did not require NIV at baseline but had symptoms in the first month of life.[37] All children in the high dose cohort were alive without the need for permanent ventilation up to 6 years after dosing.[38]

The open-label, single-arm, phase 3 trials, STR1VE-EU and STR1VE-US, showed improvement in functional independent sitting at 18 months of age in symptomatic children with SMA type 1 (1 or 2 SMN2 copies) less than 6 months of age.[39,40] In addition, 31 of 32 (97%) and 20 of 22 (91%) patients survived free from permanent ventilatory support at age 14 months in the STR1VE-EU and the STR1VE-US trials, respectively.[39,40]

The phase 3, single-arm SPR1NT trial treated presymptomatic infants (2 SMN2 copies = 14; 3 SMN2 copies = 15) with onasemnogene abeparvovec within 6 postnatal weeks. In the 3 SMN2 copy cohort, all infants stood independently before 24 months, 14 of 15 (93%) walked independently, and all survived without nutritional or respiratory support at 14 months.[41] In the 2 SMN2 copy cohort, all infants sat independently before 18 months, 10 of 14 (71%) walked independently, and all survived without nutritional or respiratory support at 14 months.[42]

Studies evaluating ventilatory requirements in children with early-onset SMA have generally found stable or improved ventilatory status following onasemnogene abeparvovec administration, with a few observational studies reporting the ability for children to completely wean off ventilation.[43,44] A minority of children are reported to develop ventilator dependence over time, particularly patients who are symptomatic with weakness within the first month of life.[11,37,43,45]

Limited data exist with respect to objective longitudinal respiratory outcomes in patients with SMA treated with onasemnogene abeparvovec. A cross-sectional study found a wide range in AHI from 3.6 to 24.1 events/hour (at 2.3–16 months of life) in 8 infants who received gene replacement therapy at 20 to 257 days of life (2 SMN2 copies = 5; 3 SMN2 copies = 2; 4 SMN2 copies = 1).[46] Another study in 11 children post-gene replacement therapy (2 SMN2 copies = 9; 3 SMN2 copies = 2) reported a range in AHI (at a median age of 22 months) from 0.2 to 8.7 events/hour.[44] Chiang and colleagues evaluated the longitudinal PSG outcomes of 11 infants with SMA identified by newborn screening (2 SMN2 copies = 7; 3

SMN2 copies = 4) who received onasemnogene abeparvovec at a median age of 3.6 weeks (5 had nusinersen pretreatment).[11] Children in this cohort had reduced sleep-disordered breathing at 1 year of life compared to natural history cohorts.[11] Two infants were prescribed nocturnal NIV for clinical respiratory symptoms and both were symptomatic with weakness at the time of onasemnogene abeparvovec administration.[11] Longer term outcomes remain to be elucidated.

Onasemnogene abeparvovec for later onset spinal muscular atrophy

Intravenous onasemnogene abeparvovec is currently unavailable for older children due to safety concerns about the maximum absolute doses that can be safely delivered. Fixed-dose intrathecal administration of onasemnogene abeparvovec may be a safe and efficacious alternative,[47] but respiratory outcomes are currently unknown.

Risdiplam

Risdiplam is an SMN2 pre-mRNA splicing modifier and the first oral drug approved for the treatment of SMA.

Risdiplam for early-onset spinal muscular atrophy

The FIREFISH clinical trial enrolled symptomatic infants with SMA and 2 SMN2 gene copies aged 1 to 7 months.[48] The primary endpoint in the second part of the 2 part study showed that 12 of 41 infants (29%) with SMA type 1 were able to sit unsupported after 12 months of therapy as compared to 0% of controls in a natural history cohort.[49] Thirty-five infants (85%) survived without permanent ventilation as compared with 42% in a natural history cohort.[49] After 24 months of treatment, 18 infants (44%) were able to sit unsupported but no infants could stand alone or walk alone.[50] One additional infant required permanent ventilation between months 12 and 24; therefore, the event-free survival at month 24 was 34 infants (83%).[50]

Risdiplam for later onset spinal muscular atrophy

The second part of the phase 3, double-blind, placebo-controlled SUNFISH clinical trial in 2 to 25 year old individuals with SMA types 2 and 3 (SMA type 2 = 120, SMA type 3 = 60) showed a significant treatment difference in the change from baseline in 32 item motor function measure (1.55; 95% CI 0.30–2.81; P = .016) in favor of risdiplam.[51] However, there were no significant differences in pulmonary function.[51] The open-label extension showed further improvement or stabilization in motor function but no improvement in

respiratory function compared to natural history findings.[52] Two small studies also reported spirometry outcomes in people using risdiplam and similarly did not find significant changes from baseline.[53,54]

SUMMARY

Aside from one study that demonstrated a slower rate of decline in percent predicted FVC during the first year of nusinersen therapy in children with SMA type 2, there is no evidence that the late initiation of nusinersen or risdiplam alter spirometry measures in symptomatic children and adults with later onset SMA. This has been attributed to irreversible chest wall restriction and contractures that develop in response to chronic chest wall muscle weakness, highlighting the importance of ongoing respiratory surveillance and treatments for people with later onset SMA receiving disease-modifying therapies.

In contrast, the initiation of disease-modifying therapies for presymptomatic infants with early-onset SMA reduces ventilation dependence and may improve sleep-disordered breathing. Further research with larger sample sizes and longer term follow-up are required.

DUCHENNE MUSCULAR DYSTROPHY

DMD is an X-linked recessive NMD caused by a mutation of the dystrophin gene, which encodes a protein that stabilizes cell membranes. The reduction in dystrophin protein results in the progressive degeneration of skeletal and cardiac muscle, leading to the loss of ambulation by 13 years of age, as well as progressive cardiomyopathy. Even with the use of corticosteroids, progression to cardiac and/or respiratory failure typically leads to death in the late twenties.[1]

Thousands of genetic mutations have been identified in the DMD gene.[55] Disease-modifying therapies target these mutations to restore dystrophin production and function.

Pulmonary Function in a Natural History Cohort

In people with DMD, skeletal muscle fiber degeneration leads to a restrictive respiratory pattern reflected by the FVC. Mayer and colleagues reported the prospective spirometry data from 60 patients with DMD aged 5.0 to 24.1 years (median age 10.3 years, 45% treated with steroids, 63.3% ambulatory at their first visit).[56] The authors demonstrated that absolute FVC and peak expiratory flow (PEF) linearly increase up to age 10 years, stabilize between 10 and 18 years, and then rapidly decline.[56] However, percent predicted FVC and PEF both declined linearly from 6 to 22 years of age with a mean (standard error [SE]) annual rate of change for percent predicted FVC and PEF of $-5.0 \pm 0.7\%$/year and $-5.8 \pm 0.6\%$/year, respectively.[56] The use of steroids has been associated with stabilization of percent predicted FVC,[57] but this is not a consistent finding.[56]

DISEASE-MODIFYING THERAPIES FOR DUCHENNE MUSCULAR DYSTROPHY
Ataluren

Approximately 10% of DMD cases are caused by nonsense mutations.[55] Ataluren is an orally bioavailable small molecule that induces ribosomal read through of nonsense mutations and partially restores dystrophin production. Ataluren has conditional approval from the European Medicines Agency but has not been approved by the FDA.

A double-blind, placebo-controlled trial in 174 boys with DMD ≥ 5 year old evaluated ataluren doses of 40 mg/kg/day and 80 mg/kg/day.[58] Although the primary endpoint of a change in 6 minute walk distance (6MWD) at week 48 was not statistically significant, there was evidence that a subgroup of patients (7–16 years of age with baseline 6MWD ≥ 150 m and <80% predicted) experienced benefit from ataluren 40 mg/kg/day.[58] A subsequent phase 3, double-blind, placebo-controlled, randomized trial was conducted in participants with similar characteristics to this subgroup and did not show a significantly different 6MWD with ataluren (difference 13.0 m; 95% CI -7.4–33.4; $P = .213$).[59] However, there was a significant effect of ataluren on a prespecified subgroup of patients with a baseline 6MWD of 300 to 400 m (difference 42.9 m; 95% CI 11.8–74.0; $P = .007$) but not in the group with a baseline 6MWD of less than 300 m or in the group with 400 m or more.[59]

A phase 3, long-term, open-label study of ataluren efficacy enrolled patients with DMD aged 2 to 28 years receiving ataluren 40 mg/kg/day and compared their results to an external natural history cohort receiving standard of care alone.[60] Using a propensity score-matched analysis, ataluren was associated with a 2.2 year delay in loss of ambulation ($P = .0006$) and a 3.0 year delay in decline of predicted FVC less than 60% in nonambulatory patients ($P = .0004$).[60] A retrospective study of ataluren in 11 patients with DMD (ataluren started at a median age of 8.4 years and followed to a median age of 16.2 years) reported that ambulatory patients increased their percent predicted FVC by a range of 2.8% to 8.2% annually, whereas

5 of 6 nonambulatory patients had an annual rate of decline in predicted FVC ranging from 1.8% to 21.1%.[61] Two of the 11 patients required nocturnal NIV by the end of the study.[61]

Exon Skipping Agents

Exon skipping refers to the use of synthetic antisense oligonucleotides to restore partially functional dystrophin protein.[62] These agents work by inducing exon skipping of problematic regions of the dystrophin gene to restore the downstream reading frame. This treatment approach is mutation-dependent and individual treatments are applicable to a small subset of individuals with DMD. However, collectively, the exon skipping strategy may treat approximately 55% of individuals with DMD.[55]

There are 4 exon skipping agents that are currently FDA-approved including eteplirsen (Exondys 51), golodirsen (Vyondys 53), viltolarsen (Viltepso), and casimersen (Amondys 45). These are delivered as once weekly intravenous infusions and have been studied as adjunct treatments to corticosteroids.

Exon 51 skipping therapy

Exon 51 skipping is applicable to approximately 14% of individuals with DMD.[55] Eteplirsen is an exon 51 skipping agent that slows the progression of DMD compared to control groups. Most evidence on eteplirsen comes from a randomized controlled trial of boys with DMD aged 7 to 13 years receiving stable doses of oral corticosteroids who were randomized to 1 of 3 arms: eteplirsen 30 mg/kg/week, eteplirsen 50 mg/kg/week, or placebo for 24 weeks.[63] Participants were followed in an open-label extension phase during which participants initially randomized to placebo were randomized to eteplirsen 30 or 50 mg/kg/week, while all other participants remained on their original dose of eteplirsen.[63] Eteplirsen was found to restore dystrophin as well as 6MWD at 48 weeks.[63] Eteplirsen-treated patients had a slower rate of decline in ambulatory function after 3 to 4 years (159 m difference between eteplirsen group and historical controls after 4 years; 95% CI 66–253 m; $P = .002$).[64] Compared to natural history studies, the eteplirsen group also appeared to have an attenuated decline in percent predicted maximal inspiratory pressure (MIP), maximal expiratory pressure (MEP), and FVC.[63,65] Specifically, the percent predicted FVC declined by 2.3% annually, which is half of expected in a natural history cohort.[65] These results persisted after a median of 6 years, at which point the change in percent predicted FVC was -3.3% compared to -6.0% in a natural history cohort

$(P < .0001).$[66] These findings have been replicated in multiple other analyses in separate cohorts of both ambulatory and nonambulatory patients.[67–69]

Exon 53 skipping therapy

Approximately 8% of individuals with DMD have mutations that can be treated with the skipping of exon 53.[55] Golodirsen and viltolarsen are the 2 exon 53 skipping therapies that have currently been FDA-approved.

Golodirsen was evaluated in a 2 part randomized, double-blind, placebo-controlled trial of boys with DMD aged 6 to 15 years. Part 1 was a dose titration study in 12 individuals with DMD (golodirsen = 8; placebo = 4) over 12 weeks and showed that golodirsen was well-tolerated.[70] Part 2 was a 168-week, open-label evaluation that found golodirsen-treated patients had an attenuated deterioration in 6MWD compared to matched exon 53 skip-amenable natural history controls after 3 years (mean difference 82.4 m; $P = .067$; $n = 25$).[71] The percent predicted FVC declined by 8.4% over 3 years of treatment, from 92.7% at baseline to 83.8% at week 144.[71]

Viltolarsen was evaluated in a phase 2, 4 week randomized clinical trial for safety followed by a 20 week open-label treatment period in patients aged 4 to 9 year old. Participants ($n = 16$, mean age 7.4 years) received high or low dose viltolarsen by weekly intravenous infusions.[72] After 20 to 24 weeks of treatment, there were significant increases in dystrophin production in both dose cohorts, and all participants showed improvements in timed function tests from baseline compared to age-matched natural history controls, including 6MWD (viltolarsen: 28.9 m; control: −65.3 m).[72] The 4 year long-term extension study found an attenuated rate of motor disease progression in viltolarsen-treated patients compared with an historical control group.[73]

Exon 45 skipping therapy

Approximately 9% of individuals with DMD have mutations that can be treated with the skipping of exon 45.[55] Casimersen was approved under FDAs accelerated approval program and the interim results from an ongoing, double-blind, placebo-controlled, randomized clinical trial (NCT02500381) showed that casimersen resulted in increased dystrophin after 48 weeks.[74]

Gene Transfer Therapy

Gene transfer therapy is a promising molecular approach for muscle fiber rescue before fiber loss. Delandistrogene moxeparvovec-rokl, a microdystrophin transgene delivered by a 1 time intravenous infusion, is the first gene therapy approved by the FDA for boys with DMD aged 4 to 5 years.[75] A nonrandomized controlled trial in 4 patients found few adverse events associated with therapy administration.[76] A larger double-blind, placebo-controlled, randomized controlled trial in 41 boys with DMD aged 4 to 7 year old has been conducted (NCT03769116). The trial evaluated the expression of microdystrophin in skeletal muscle at week 12 as well as the change in North Star Ambulatory Assessment (NSAA) total score from baseline to week 48. Although the difference between the overall treatment and placebo groups was not statistically significant for the NSAA total score at week 48, a post hoc exploratory subgroup analysis suggested benefit in subjects aged 4 to 5 years (mean change [SE] in NSAA total score from baseline to week 48 was 4.3 [0.7] points for the treatment group versus 1.9 [0.7] points for the placebo group).[75] Additional trials are currently underway.

Summary

Respiratory outcomes with disease-modifying therapies in DMD are largely unknown. The available trial data for the exon skipping agents, eteplirsen and golodirsen, suggest that these therapies may reduce the rate of percent predicted FVC decline. Reduced rates of decline in percent predicted FVC have also been described following ataluren administration, but only in nonrandomized studies.

FUTURE DIRECTIONS

Respiratory outcomes with disease-modifying therapies are typically derived from small studies. This highlights the need for larger, multicenter studies to provide in-depth knowledge about disease-modifying therapy impact on respiratory function. Longitudinal studies following patients over longer periods of time may also elucidate potential side effects and long-term effects. Further studies among diverse populations should evaluate predictors for treatment response to inform therapy decision-making. Specifically, the phenotyping of SMA and DMD may help to tailor appropriate therapy. Additionally, health economic studies evaluating these expensive disease-modifying therapies may inform public policy and ensure equitable access to therapy.

Many clinical trials in infants with SMA include the endpoint of permanent ventilatory assistance as a component of a composite primary outcome. However, indications for ventilation are not standardized and may be at the discretion of the clinical team as one aspect of a larger proactive treatment approach. Although PSG data may provide important respiratory function data for these patients, infant PSGs are burdensome and not widely available. As such, future research to evaluate sensitive respiratory function outcomes for infants and young children with SMA is essential to inform suitable respiratory endpoints in future clinical trials.

SUMMARY

The current landscape of care for patients with SMA and DMD is rapidly shifting as increasing numbers of disease-modifying therapies become widely available. Although respiratory failure is one of the leading causes of death in people with SMA and DMD, respiratory outcome data associated with disease-modifying therapies are sparse. Available data suggest that novel therapeutics attenuate the natural trajectory of respiratory decline but do not reverse disease. It is therefore of great importance that ongoing respiratory surveillance and monitoring are integrated in the care of people with NMD on disease-modifying therapies.

CLINICS CARE POINTS

- Disease-modifying therapies for SMA and DMD are rapidly shifting current paradigms of care.
- Disease-modifying therapies generally attenuate the natural trajectory of respiratory decline but do not reverse disease.
- Ongoing respiratory surveillance and monitoring are an integral component of care for people on disease-modifying therapies.

DISCLOSURE

Dr R. Amin is a committee member of the American College of Chest Physicians and a pediatrics committee member of the American Thoracic Society. R. Amin holds research grants from Canadian Institutes of Health Research, Canada, Cure SMA Canada, Canada, Muscular Dystrophy Canada, Canada, VHA Home Healthcare, Canada, Boehringer-Ingelheim, Germany, Medigas, Canada, ProResp, Canada, Baxter Corporation Endowment Fund for Home Care, United States, and Ontario Ministry of Health and Long-Term Care, Canada. Dr L. Xiao is a committee member of the American College of Chest Physicians. Dr. Xiao holds research grants from Muscular Dystrophy Canada, Baxter Corporation Endowment Fund for Home Care, International Pediatric Sleep Association, United States, and the Sleep Research Society Foundation, United States.

REFERENCES

1. Passamano L, Taglia A, Palladino A, et al. Improvement of survival in duchenne muscular dystrophy: retrospective analysis of 835 patients. Acta Myol 2012;31(2):121–5.
2. Rall S, Grimm T. Survival in Duchenne muscular dystrophy. Acta Myol 2012;31(2):117–20.
3. Lefebvre S, Bürglen L, Reboullet S, et al. Identification and characterization of a spinal muscular atrophy-determining gene. Cell 1995;80(1):155–65.
4. Kolb SJ, Coffey CS, Yankey JW, et al. Natural history of infantile-onset spinal muscular atrophy. Ann Neurol 2017;82(6):883–91.
5. Gregoretti C, Ottonello G, Chiarini Testa MB, et al. Survival of patients with spinal muscular atrophy type 1. Pediatrics 2013;131(5):e1509–14.
6. Finkel RS, McDermott MP, Kaufmann P, et al. Observational study of spinal muscular atrophy type I and implications for clinical trials. Neurology 2014;83(9): 810–7.
7. Kapur N, Deegan S, Parakh A, et al. Relationship between respiratory function and need for NIV in childhood SMA. Pediatr Pulmonol 2019;54(11): 1774–80.
8. Wijngaarde CA, Veldhoen ES, Van Eijk RPA, et al. Natural history of lung function in spinal muscular atrophy. Orphanet J Rare Dis 2020;15(1):88.
9. Trucco F, Ridout D, Scoto M, et al. Respiratory trajectories in type 2 and 3 spinal muscular atrophy in the iSMAC cohort study. Neurology 2021;96(4): e587–99.
10. Chacko A, Sly PD, Gauld L. Polysomnography findings in pediatric spinal muscular atrophy types 1–3. Sleep Med 2020;68:124–30.
11. Chiang J, Xiao L, Nigro E, et al. Sleep disordered breathing in infants identified through newborn screening with spinal muscular atrophy. Sleep Med 2023;111:161–9.
12. Hua Y, Sahashi K, Hung G, et al. Antisense correction of SMN2 splicing in the CNS rescues necrosis in a type III SMA mouse model. Genes Dev 2010; 24(15):1634–44.
13. Finkel RS, Mercuri E, Darras BT, et al. Nusinersen versus sham control in infantile-onset spinal muscular atrophy. N Engl J Med 2017;377(18):1723–32.
14. Crawford TO, Swoboda KJ, De Vivo DC, et al. Continued benefit of nusinersen initiated in the presymptomatic stage of spinal muscular atrophy: 5-year update of the NURTURE study. Muscle Nerve 2023;68(2):157–70.
15. De Vivo DC, Bertini E, Swoboda KJ, et al. Nusinersen initiated in infants during the presymptomatic

stage of spinal muscular atrophy: interim efficacy and safety results from the Phase 2 NURTURE study. Neuromuscul Disord 2019;29(11):842–56.

16. Lavie M, Diamant N, Cahal M, et al. Nusinersen for spinal muscular atrophy type 1: real-world respiratory experience. Pediatr Pulmonol 2021;56:291–8.

17. Sansone VA, Pirola A, Albamonte E, et al. Respiratory needs in patients with type 1 spinal muscular atrophy treated with nusinersen. J Pediatr 2020;219: 223–8.

18. Pechmann A, Langer T, Schorling D, et al. Evaluation of children with SMA type 1 under treatment with nusinersen within the expanded access program in Germany. J Neuromuscul Dis 2018;5(2):135–43.

19. Chen KA, Widger J, Teng A, et al. Real-world respiratory and bulbar comorbidities of SMA type 1 children treated with nusinersen: 2-Year single centre Australian experience. Paediatr Respir Rev 2020; 39:54–60.

20. Farrar MA, Teoh HL, Carey KA, et al. Nusinersen for SMA: expanded access programme. J Neurol Neurosurg Psychiatry 2018;89(9):937–42.

21. Xiao L, Chiang J, Castro-Codesal M, et al. Respiratory characteristics in children with spinal muscular atrophy type 1 receiving nusinersen. Pediatr Pulmonol 2022;58(1):161–70.

22. Chacko A, Sly PD, Ware RS, et al. Effect of nusinersen on respiratory function in paediatric spinal muscular atrophy types 1–3. Thorax 2022;77:40–6.

23. Aragon-Gawinska K, Seferian AM, Daron A, et al. Nusinersen in patients older than 7 months with spinal muscular atrophy type 1: a cohort study. Neurology 2018;91(14):e1312–8.

24. Panagiotou P, Kanaka-Gantenbein C, Kaditis AG. Changes in ventilatory support requirements of spinal muscular atrophy (SMA) patients post gene-based therapies. Children 2022;9(8):1207.

25. Pechmann A, Behrens M, Dörnbrack K, et al. Effect of nusinersen on motor, respiratory and bulbar function in early-onset spinal muscular atrophy. Brain 2023;146(2):668–77.

26. Pane M, Coratti G, Sansone VA, et al. Type I spinal muscular atrophy patients treated with nusinersen: 4-year follow-up of motor, respiratory and bulbar function. Euro J of Neurology 2023;30(6):1755–63.

27. Hepkaya E, Kılınç Sakallı AA, Ülkersoy İ, et al. The effects of nusinersen treatment on respiratory status of children with spinal muscular atrophy. Pediatr Int 2022;64(1):e15310.

28. Scheijmans FEV, Cuppen I, Van Eijk RPA, et al. Population-based assessment of nusinersen efficacy in children with spinal muscular atrophy: a 3-year follow-up study. Brain Communications 2022;4(6): fcac269.

29. Tscherter A, Rüsch CT, Baumann D, et al. Evaluation of real-life outcome data of patients with spinal muscular atrophy treated with nusinersen in

Switzerland. Neuromuscul Disord 2022;32(5): 399–409.

30. Mercuri E, Darras BT, Chiriboga CA, et al. Nusinersen versus sham control in later-onset spinal muscular atrophy. N Engl J Med 2018;378(7): 625–35.

31. Acsadi G, Crawford TO, Müller-Felber W, et al. Safety and efficacy of nusinersen in spinal muscular atrophy: the EMBRACE study. Muscle Nerve 2021; 63(5):668–77.

32. Gonski K, Chuang S, Teng A, et al. Respiratory and sleep outcomes in children with SMA treated with nusinersen - real world experience. Neuromuscul Disord 2023;33(6):531–8.

33. Heitschmidt L, Pichlmaier L, Eckerland M, et al. Nusinersen does not improve lung function in a cohort of children with spinal muscular atrophy – a single-center retrospective study. Eur J Paediatr Neurol 2021;31:88–91.

34. Fainmesser Y, Drory VE, Ben-Shushan S, et al. Longer-term follow-up of nusinersen efficacy and safety in adult patients with spinal muscular atrophy types 2 and 3. Neuromuscul Disord 2022;32(6):451–9.

35. Elsheikh B, Severyn S, Zhao S, et al. Safety, tolerability, and effect of nusinersen in non-ambulatory adults with spinal muscular atrophy. Front Neurol 2021;12:650532.

36. Mendell JR, Al-Zaidy S, Shell R, et al. Single-dose gene-replacement therapy for spinal muscular atrophy. N Engl J Med 2017;377(18):1713–22.

37. Al-Zaidy S, Pickard AS, Kotha K, et al. Health outcomes in spinal muscular atrophy type 1 following AVXS-101 gene replacement therapy. Pediatr Pulmonol 2019;54(2):179–85.

38. Mendell JR, Al-Zaidy SA, Lehman KJ, et al. Five-year extension results of the phase 1 start trial of onasemnogene abeparvovec in spinal muscular atrophy. JAMA Neurol 2021;78(7):834.

39. Mercuri E, Muntoni F, Baranello G, et al. Onasemnogene abeparvovec gene therapy for symptomatic infantile-onset spinal muscular atrophy type 1 (STR1VE-EU): an open-label, single-arm, multicentre, phase 3 trial. Lancet Neurol 2021;20(10): 832–41.

40. Day JW, Finkel RS, Chiriboga CA, et al. Onasemnogene abeparvovec gene therapy for symptomatic infantile-onset spinal muscular atrophy in patients with two copies of SMN2 (STR1VE): an open-label, single-arm, multicentre, phase 3 trial. Lancet Neurol 2021;20(4):284–93.

41. Strauss KA, Farrar MA, Muntoni F, et al. Onasemnogene abeparvovec for presymptomatic infants with three copies of SMN2 at risk for spinal muscular atrophy: the Phase III SPR1NT trial. Nat Med 2022; 28(7):1390–7.

42. Strauss KA, Farrar MA, Muntoni F, et al. Onasemnogene abeparvovec for presymptomatic infants with

two copies of SMN2 at risk for spinal muscular atrophy type 1: the Phase III SPR1NT trial. Nat Med 2022;28(7):1381–9.

43. D'Silva AM, Holland S, Kariyawasam D, et al. Onasemnogene abeparvovec in spinal muscular atrophy: an Australian experience of safety and efficacy. Ann Clin Transl Neurol 2022;9(3):339–50.

44. AlNaimi A, Hamad SG, Mohamed RBA, et al. A breakthrough effect of gene replacement therapy on respiratory outcomes in children with spinal muscular atrophy. Pediatr Pulmonol 2023;58(4):1004–11.

45. Stettner GM, Hasselmann O, Tscherter A, et al. Treatment of spinal muscular atrophy with Onasemnogene Abeparvovec in Switzerland: a prospective observational case series study. BMC Neurol 2023;23(1):88.

46. Leon-Astudillo C, Wagner M, Salabarria SM, et al. Polysomnography findings in children with spinal muscular atrophy after onasemnogene-abeparvovec. Sleep Med 2023;101:234–7.

47. Finkel RS, Darras BT, Mendell JR, et al. Intrathecal onasemnogene abeparvovec for sitting, nonambulatory patients with spinal muscular atrophy: phase i ascending-dose study (STRONG). JND 2023;10(3):389–404.

48. Baranello G, Darras BT, Day JW, et al. Risdiplam in type 1 spinal muscular atrophy. N Engl J Med 2021;384(10):915–23.

49. Darras BT, Masson R, Mazurkiewicz-Bełdzińska M, et al. Risdiplam-treated infants with type 1 spinal muscular atrophy versus historical controls. N Engl J Med 2021;385(5):427–35.

50. Masson R, Mazurkiewicz-Bełdzińska M, Rose K, et al. Safety and efficacy of risdiplam in patients with type 1 spinal muscular atrophy (FIREFISH part 2): secondary analyses from an open-label trial. Lancet Neurol 2022;21(12):1110–9.

51. Mercuri E, Deconinck N, Mazzone ES, et al. Safety and efficacy of once-daily risdiplam in type 2 and non-ambulant type 3 spinal muscular atrophy (SUNFISH part 2): a phase 3, double-blind, randomised, placebo-controlled trial. Lancet Neurol 2022;21(1):42–52.

52. Oskoui M, Day JW, Deconinck N, et al. Two-year efficacy and safety of risdiplam in patients with type 2 or non-ambulant type 3 spinal muscular atrophy (SMA). J Neurol 2023;270(5):2531–46.

53. McCluskey G, Lamb S, Mason S, et al. Risdiplam for the treatment of adults with spinal muscular atrophy: experience of the Northern Ireland neuromuscular service. Muscle Nerve 2023;67(2):157–61.

54. Ñungo Garzón NC, Pitarch Castellano I, Sevilla T, et al. Risdiplam in non-sitter patients aged 16 years and older with 5q spinal muscular atrophy. Muscle Nerve 2023;67(5):407–11.

55. Bladen CL, Salgado D, Monges S, et al. The TREAT-NMD DMD global database: analysis of more than 7,000 duchenne muscular dystrophy mutations. Hum Mutat 2015;36(4):395–402.

56. Mayer OH, Finkel RS, Rummey C, et al. Characterization of pulmonary function in duchenne muscular dystrophy. Pediatr Pulmonol 2015;50(5):487–94.

57. Biggar WD, Gingras M, Fehlings DL, et al. Deflazacort treatment of Duchenne muscular dystrophy. J Pediatr 2001;138(1):45–50.

58. Bushby K, Finkel R, Wong B, et al. Ataluren treatment of patients with nonsense mutation dystrophinopathy. Muscle Nerve 2014;50(4):477–87.

59. McDonald CM, Campbell C, Torricelli RE, et al. Ataluren in patients with nonsense mutation Duchenne muscular dystrophy (ACT DMD): a multicentre, randomised, double-blind, placebo-controlled, phase 3 trial. Lancet 2017;390(10101):1489–98.

60. McDonald CM, Muntoni F, Penematsa V, et al. Ataluren delays loss of ambulation and respiratory decline in nonsense mutation Duchenne muscular dystrophy patients. J Comp Eff Res 2022;11(3):139–55.

61. Michael E, Sofou K, Wahlgren L, et al. Long term treatment with ataluren—the Swedish experience. BMC Musculoskelet Disord 2021;22(1):837.

62. Mann CJ, Honeyman K, Cheng AJ, et al. Antisense-induced exon skipping and synthesis of dystrophin in the mdx mouse. Proc Natl Acad Sci U S A 2001;98(1):42–7.

63. Mendell JR, Goemans N, Lowes LP, et al. Longitudinal effect of eteplirsen versus historical control on ambulation in Duchenne muscular dystrophy. Ann Neurol 2016;79(2):257–71.

64. Mendell JR, Khan N, Sha N, et al. Comparison of long-term ambulatory function in patients with duchenne muscular dystrophy treated with eteplirsen and matched natural history controls. JND 2021;8(4):469–79.

65. Kinane TB, Mayer OH, Duda PW, et al. Long-term pulmonary function in duchenne muscular dystrophy: comparison of eteplirsen-treated patients to natural history. JND 2018;5(1):47–58.

66. Mitelman O, Abdel-Hamid HZ, Byrne BJ, et al. A combined prospective and retrospective comparison of long-term functional outcomes suggests delayed loss of ambulation and pulmonary decline with long-term eteplirsen treatment. JND 2022;9(1):39–52.

67. Khan N, Eliopoulos H, Han L, et al. Eteplirsen treatment attenuates respiratory decline in ambulatory and non-ambulatory patients with duchenne muscular dystrophy. JND 2019;6(2):213–25.

68. Iff J, Gerrits C, Zhong Y, et al. Delays in pulmonary decline in eteplirsen-treated patients with Duchenne muscular dystrophy. Muscle Nerve 2022;66(3):262–9.

69. McDonald CM, Shieh PB, Abdel-Hamid HZ, et al. Open-label evaluation of eteplirsen in patients with duchenne muscular dystrophy amenable to exon 51 skipping: PROMOVI trial. JND 2021;8(6): 989–1001.

70. Frank DE, Schnell FJ, Akana C, et al. Increased dystrophin production with golodirsen in patients with Duchenne muscular dystrophy. Neurology 2020; 94(21):e2270–82.

71. Servais L, Mercuri E, Straub V, et al. Long-term safety and efficacy data of golodirsen in ambulatory patients with duchenne muscular dystrophy amenable to exon 53 skipping: a first-in-human, multicenter, two-part, open-label, phase 1/2 trial. Nucleic Acid Therapeut 2022;32(1):29–39.

72. Clemens PR, Rao VK, Connolly AM, et al. Safety, tolerability, and efficacy of viltolarsen in boys with duchenne muscular dystrophy amenable to exon 53 skipping: a phase 2 randomized clinical trial. JAMA Neurol 2020;77(8):982.

73. Clemens PR, Rao VK, Connolly AM, et al. Efficacy and safety of viltolarsen in boys with duchenne muscular dystrophy: results from the phase 2, open-label, 4-year extension study. JND 2023; 10(3):439–47.

74. US FDA. Amondys 45 (casimersen) injection, for intravenous use. US prescribing information; 2021. Available at: https://www.accessdata.fda.gov/drugsatfda_docs/label/2021/213026lbl.pdf. [Accessed 23 October 2023].

75. US FDA. Elevidys (delandistrogene moxeparvovec-rokl): summary basis for regulatory action. 2023. Available at: https://www.fda.gov/media/169746/download?attachment. [Accessed 23 October 2023].

76. Mendell JR, Sahenk Z, Lehman K, et al. Assessment of systemic delivery of rAAVrh74.MHCK7.microdystrophin in children with duchenne muscular dystrophy: a nonrandomized controlled trial. JAMA Neurol 2020;77(9):1122.

Airway Clearance in Neuromuscular Disease

Nicole L. Sheers, BPhysio(Hons), MPhysio, PhD[a,b,*], Tiina Andersen, BSc(Hons), MSc, PhD[c,d], Michelle Chatwin, BSc(Hons), PhD[e,f]

KEYWORDS

- Physiotherapy • Duchenne muscular dystrophy • Amyotrophic lateral sclerosis
- Mechanical insufflation-exsufflation (MI-E) • Cough assist • Lung volume recruitment (LVR)

KEY POINTS

- The respiratory management of people with neuromuscular disease (pwNMD) should include an assessment of cough and the ability to clear secretions.
- In pwNMD who have bulbar involvement, the efficacy of mechanical insufflation-exsufflation therapy should be further evaluated, either with auscultation of the trachea, transnasal fiberoptic laryngoscopy, or graphical analysis, to ensure effective treatment.
- There is a role for hyperinflation therapies in pwNMD, for cough augmentation and possibly thoracic range of motion. Treatment should be personalized to the individual.
- pwNMD who have recurrent respiratory exacerbations despite optimal proximal airway clearance techniques should be started on a peripheral airway clearance regime and evaluated for chronic suppurative lung disease.

INTRODUCTION

Hypoventilation and chronic hypercapnic respiratory failure are common sequelae of many neuromuscular diseases (NMD) where respiratory muscle weakness is a feature, including amyotrophic lateral sclerosis (ALS), spinal muscular atrophy (SMA), Duchenne muscular dystrophy (DMD), and other genetic myopathies. Cough function is often impaired, and is further compromised in the event of an upper or lower respiratory tract infection (RTI).[1] In some people with NMD (pwNMD), bulbar insufficiency leads to difficulty managing saliva, clearing secretions from the mouth, and aspiration. Poor management of oral secretions can lead to poor tolerance of respiratory support techniques.[2]

Multiple guidelines advocate the use of noninvasive ventilation (NIV) to improve hypoventilation-related symptoms, awake hypercapnia, quality of life, and reduce the risk of unplanned hospitalization and mortality.[3–10] Increasingly, airway clearance techniques (ACTs) are recognized as an integral component of the multi-perspective and multidisciplinary respiratory management of NMDs, to help clear mucus from the lungs and improve breathing.[11–13] Secretion location guides treatment, with the principles being to (i) open up the airways and get air behind mucus, (ii) loosen/unstick secretions from the small airways, (iii) mobilize secretions through the airways to the larger airways, and (iv) clear secretions from the central airways, usually with a cough.[14]

[a] Department of Physiotherapy, Melbourne School of Health Sciences, The University of Melbourne, Parkville, Victoria, Australia; [b] The Institute for Breathing and Sleep, Austin Health, Heidelberg, Victoria, Australia; [c] The Department of Health and Functioning, Western Norway University of Applied Science, Postboks 7030, 5020 Bergen, Norway; [d] Thoracic Department, Haukeland University Hospital, Postboks 1400, 5021 Bergen, Norway; [e] NMCC, The National Hospital for Neurology and Neurosurgery, University College London Hospitals Foundation Trust, London WC1N 3BG, UK; [f] Clinical and Academic Department of Sleep and Breathing, Royal Brompton Hospital, Part of Guys and St Thomas' NHS Foundation Trust, London SW3 6NP, UK
* Corresponding author. Institute for Breathing and Sleep, Austin Health, 145 Studley Road, Heidelberg, Victoria, Australia 3084.
E-mail address: nsheers@unimelb.edu.au

Sleep Med Clin 19 (2024) 485–496
https://doi.org/10.1016/j.jsmc.2024.04.009
1556-407X/24/© 2024 Elsevier Inc. All rights reserved.

Guidelines incorporating ACTs are largely consensus-based due to the low to very low certainty of evidence for interventions.[3] A 2017 European Neuromuscular Center (ENMC) international workshop highlighted the gap between the science and clinical practice of ACTs in NMDs, emphasized the critical role of expert consensus opinions due to the lack of controlled clinical research, and developed universally applicable recommendations for pwNMD, noting that "absence of evidence of benefit is not evidence of absence of benefit."[11] An algorithmic approach to treatment was devised, comprising ventilatory/medical support and ACT management. "Peripheral ACTs" encompass therapies aimed at mobilizing secretions (eg, manual techniques, high-frequency chest wall oscillation [HFCWO], intrapulmonary percussive ventilation [IPV], chest wall strapping), whereas those that clear the central airways were categorized as "proximal ACTs" (eg, manually assisted cough [MAC], glossopharyngeal breathing [GPB], single and stacked breath-assisted inspiration, and mechanical insufflation-exsufflation [MI-E]).[11,12] Cough peak flow (CPF) was acknowledged as a common marker for assessing ACT effectiveness in NMDs; however, the consensus group identified the need for an internationally recognized standard for measuring CPF as a future research priority.

More recently, the American College of Chest Physicians (ACCP) addressed 9 clinical questions regarding respiratory management in NMD, including "Should ACTs be used for patients with NMD?." The guideline suggested (i) GPB be considered for volume recruitment and airway clearance when hypoventilation was present; (ii) MAC, either independently or combined with other techniques, be used when cough effectiveness was reduced; (iii) regular lung volume recruitment (LVR) be used when reduced lung function and cough effectiveness were identified; (iv) regular MI-E be used to improve cough effectiveness when alternative techniques were inadequate, and (v) HFCWO be used for secretion mobilization when difficulties with secretion clearance were present. These recommendations were noted to all have a very low certainty of evidence.[3]

New evidence regarding the effect of ACTs in pwNMD has emerged since the ENMC, ACCP, and other review papers were published. **Fig. 1** highlights additional respiratory therapy strategies in the management of pwNMD beyond the published guidelines. A greater understanding of the upper airway response to one of the most recommended ACTs, MI-E, has demonstrated the importance of individualizing titration to optimize therapy, and there is also growing knowledge of how to titrate MI-E therapy for people with ALS[15–19] and children.[20–22] Other work has shed light on the short-term effects of volume recruitment therapies during periods of stability in NMD,[23–30] as well as longer-term effects of regular therapy.[31–33] Moreover, advances in pharmacotherapies and multidisciplinary management are changing the natural history of many NMDs, meaning clinical services are seeing people living longer with chronic NMD. As survival improves, there is a greater role for ACTs and other respiratory therapies to help manage the ensuing respiratory muscle weakness and potential concomitant comorbidities

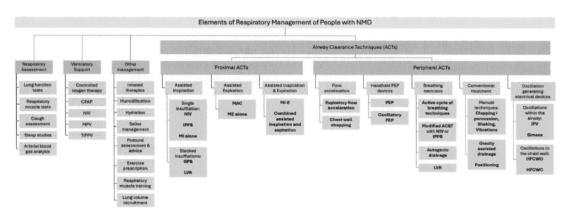

Fig. 1. Respiratory therapy strategies, including airway clearance techniques, in people living with neuromuscular disease. ACBT, active cycle of breathing technique; CPAP, continuous positive airway pressure; GPB, glossopharyngeal breathing; HFCWC, high-frequency chest well compression; HFCWO, high-frequency chest wall oscillation; IPPB, intermittent positive pressure breathing; IPV, intrapulmonary percussive ventilation; LVR, lung volume recruitment; MAC, manual assisted cough; ME, mechanical insufflation; MI, mechanical insufflation; MI-E, mechanical insufflation-exsufflation; MPV, mouthpiece ventilation; NIV, non-invasive ventilation; PEP, positive expiratory pressure; TIPPV, tracheostomy intermittent positive pressure ventilation.

(eg, dysphagia, recurrent aspiration, RTIs, chronic suppurative lung disease, and musculoskeletal abnormalities of the chest wall).

One of the challenges in treating pwNMD is that disease progression may be fast or slow and varies even within the same diagnosis. Respiratory impairment impacts on other issues and vice versa, and care strategies interact in a complex manner.[34] Whilst algorithms and recommendations can help guide management, it is imperative to provide person-centered treatment rather than treat the diagnosis. This review will focus on advances in the ACT field viewed through this problem-based approach, specifically cough assessment, individualization of MI-E, hyperinflation, and peripheral secretion mobilization techniques.

COUGH ASSESSMENT

Assessing cough is an integral element of managing pwNMD. An ineffective cough is an indication for commencing ACTs, and the degree of impairment influences technique selection.[11,12] A normal cough consists of 3 components (**Fig. 2**); however, in pwNMD, the inspiratory phase may be prolonged with a reduced peak inspiratory flow rate,

the compression phase shortened or absent, and the expiratory flow rise time may be increased with a lower expiratory CPF.[35]

The most common measure of cough in pwNMD is CPF.[36] However, this parameter measures only one component of cough. Whilst studies have documented CPF cut-off values associated with effectively clearing respiratory secretions,[37,38] other cough airflow metrics, such as compressive phase duration, peak expiratory flow rise time, cough volume acceleration, and cough expired volume (CEV), have also been identified as important for effective cough generation.[39–41] Current thinking is that weak and ineffective coughs are characterized by *at least one of* an absent cough compression phase, low CPF, CEV, and/or cough volume acceleration values. Moreover, CPF in isolation does not necessarily reflect clinician rating of cough effectiveness and strength, with strong, effective coughs seen at low CPFs and weak, ineffective coughs seen at higher CPFs.[39] Lacombe and colleagues[41] have demonstrated increasing CPF values in the presence of upper airway collapse in pwNMD using MI-E, which similarly suggests that CPF does not always reflect cough effectiveness. Mathematical modeling

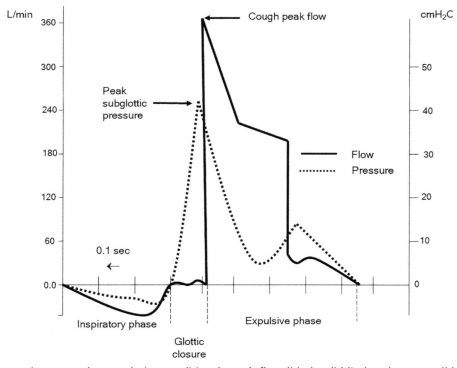

Fig. 2. Flow and pressure changes during a volitional cough flow (*black solid line*) and pressure (*black dotted line*) changes during a normal cough. Three components are illustrated: (1) inspiratory phase, (2) glottic closure (approximately 0.2 seconds duration), and (3) expiratory phase. A cough peak flow of greater than 360 L/min is considered normal.

using a 3-dimensional human airway geometry model and computational fluid dynamics has found that changing CPF has minimal effect on mucus clearance under normal and low mucus viscosity; however, increasing CEV can improve mucus clearance regardless of viscosity or thickness.[42]

Simple assessment of cough efficacy should not be forgotten. Qualitative assessment comprises (i) asking the pwNMD to assess the effectiveness of their cough when well and when unwell (ie, *Can your cough clear secretions?*), (ii) observing a volitional cough, noting rib cage and abdominal movement patterns and if secretions are cleared, and (iii) clinician rating of cough (sound, strength, perceived effectiveness, presence of secretions). If the pwNMD cannot cough to command, a spontaneous (reflex) cough might be witnessed during the consultation and can be used. However, it is important to note the type of cough assessed as the respiratory kinematic and airflow characteristics differ between the two (eg, reflex CPF lower than volitional CPF).[35,43] Auscultating the trachea may be helpful to help detect airway collapse on inspiration or expiration, and asking a patient to repeat the letter "e" can give an indication of the opening and closing of the vocal cords, allowing an opinion to be made on glottic function.

Other methods to evaluate cough are emerging. Subjective cough sound quality has previously been shown to correlate with a maximum expiratory pressure at the mouth (MEP), and a MEP of greater than 60 cmH$_2$O has been defined as the cutoff for an effective cough.[44] More recently, a smartphone app has been developed that records cough sounds and estimates the CPF ("cough peak sound", measured in L/min) based on the cough peak sound pressure level measured using the smartphone microphone (dB).[45,46] Whilst this technology shows promise as a widespread, portable method of assessing cough, it currently lacks accuracy as a 1:1 surrogate method for measuring CPF. Moreover, utility in the setting of background noise or MI-E devices should be investigated.

Currently, CPF remains the main tool for evaluating cough over time, in addition to guiding the initiation of and assessing the effect of ACTs. Many guidelines recommend commencing proximal ACTs when a CPF is less than 270 L/min,[6,7,10] and MI-E once CPF falls below 160 L/min.[10] CPF is also used to measure the effectiveness of proximal ACTs as a cough augmentation technique, by comparing the unassisted CPF to the assisted CPF value. However, it has recently been noted that CPF values during MI-E can increase in the presence of upper airway closure on either insufflation, exsufflation, or both.[19,47–49] **Fig. 3** illustrates how an MI-E device can register high expiratory flow rates due to air within the circuit rather than true cough expiratory flow.

Interpreting CPF values in clinical care requires an understanding of normal values. In healthy children, CPF does not reach more than 360 L/min until the age of 12 years;[50] hence, applying CPF cutoffs to a pediatric population is problematic. One option for children aged 12 years or younger is to use a CPF threshold based on less than fifth percentile for age.[3] Alternatively, predicted forced vital capacity (FVC) or respiratory muscle strength

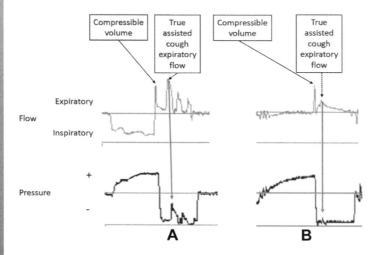

Fig. 3. Flow and pressure changes during cough with mechanical insufflation-exsufflation flow (*top panel, light blue*) and pressure (*bottom panel, dark blue*) changes during mechanical insufflation-exsufflation (MI-E), where insufflation pressure (+) and exsufflation pressure (−). Example: A represents a normal MI-E assisted cough. The first peak labeled compressible volume represents air being sucked out of the circuit prior to the opening of the upper airway. This peak may not be seen if a cough occurs at this exact time; instead a positive spike on the exsufflation pressure in conjunction with a high expiratory flow may be observed. The true assisted expiratory flow is highlighted, and the red arrow shows the corresponding positive spike on the exsufflation pressure. In example B, insufflation and exsufflation pressures are visible; however, there is little inspiratory flow indicating upper airway closure, and a concomitant reduction in expiratory flow and volume of air being delivered to the lungs.

may better indicate the severity of the cough impairment.[51] Similarly, there are little data describing the "normal" CPF value for pwNMD. Although most pwNMD may have a CPF below that of normal healthy adults, this may be within the range of normal for people living with respiratory muscle weakness and may not be pathologic. Observed CPF values differ widely within and between diseases, and the natural history and rate of progression needs to be considered when interpreting an individual's CPF value.[52,53] In one cohort of pwNMD and moderately severe respiratory system involvement, 90% of participants had a CPF below the recommended threshold for prescribing assisted cough techniques (270 L/min), yet less than half the group had experienced an RTI in the previous year.[27] Although an individual's CPF may fall below published cutoff values, other clinical factors should also be taken into account to help avoid prescribing therapies that may not be indicated.

MECHANICAL INSUFFLATION-EXSUFFLATION TITRATION

The most recommended ACT in pwNMD is MI-E. The goal of MI-E treatment is to ensure effective airway clearance while ensuring safety, comfort, and maintenance of upper airway patency. To achieve this, a personalized and patient-centered approach for titrating MI-E settings is recommended.[17,54,55] In clinical practice, an algorithm for initial MI-E titration is a helpful starting point for novice users.[54] During titration, the pwNMD's cough effort and a comprehensive assessment of measures such as CPF, vital capacity (VC), maximal inspiratory pressure, and MEP should be considered. Adjustments should be made to optimize chest wall movement during insufflation, exsufflation, and pauses. To prevent mask leakage, judicious titration of insufflation pressure and ensuring a good mask seal without pushing the jaw posteriorly are required. User involvement is essential, and feedback from the pwNMD should include whether they perceive enhanced cough effectiveness. An increase in cough audibility can serve as an additional indicator of improved cough strength.[54]

In individuals with poor laryngeal control, therapeutic positive pressures may provoke disadvantageous laryngeal responses, precluding air filling the lungs and compromising attempts to assist the expiratory phase of cough (**Fig. 3**B). This leads to inefficient MI-E therapy, discomfort, and potentially affects usage. A greater understanding of the upper airway response to MI-E has demonstrated the importance of individualizing titration to optimize therapy, especially in individuals with bulbar muscular dysfunction.[16,18,19,56]

Dynamic transnasal fiberoptic laryngoscopy assessment during ongoing MI-E therapy has proven valuable for observing laryngeal response patterns in healthy individuals and those with disease.[16,18,56–58] In healthy subjects, the larynx behaves similarly to a voluntary cough, with glottis abduction during insufflation and exsufflation, and coordinated glottic closure upon cough instruction.[57] In contrast, individuals with ALS, even those without bulbar symptoms, exhibit a brief initial abduction of the true vocal folds followed by subsequent adduction during both insufflation and exsufflation. Those without bulbar symptoms may struggle to coordinate laryngeal cough movements during rapid MI-E cycles, experiencing a backward movement of the tongue base during insufflation and hypopharyngeal constriction during exsufflation. In people with ALS and bulbar symptoms, prominent laryngeal closure during insufflation, especially at high positive pressures, is common. Therefore, vigorous insufflation is proposed as a contributing factor to the ineffectiveness of MI-E treatment.[56]

In general, the initial inspiratory airflow should not enter the upper airway too abruptly. High inspiratory pressures can induce laryngeal closure; hence, pressure adjustments should be gently titrated upwards. Reduced insufflation flows (ie, longer rise time) together with asymmetrical pressure settings (insufflation<exsufflation) can prevent laryngeal closure. Extending the inspiratory time might be necessary to attain the required insufflation volume before exsufflation. Rapid MI-E cycles are often poorly tolerated by individuals with bulbar dysfunction. Successful treatment requires a "resetting" of the larynx after exsufflation, with swallowing or closing reflexes concluding before the subsequent insufflation. A prolonged time interval between exsufflation and insufflation, or employing one cough cycle at a time, may allow the larynx to prepare for the subsequent insufflation.[18]

Direct laryngeal visualization during MI-E is the best and most objective approach to observe how the upper airway responds to treatment.[17] If this is not available, simple throat/tracheal auscultation can provide insights into laryngeal airflow and synchronization of glottic closure during MI-E cycles. By placing a stethoscope on the side of the neck near the larynx, changes in airflow during MI-E can be discerned.[59] Sancho and colleagues[19] demonstrated the utility of inspiratory and expiratory MI-E volumes in detecting upper airway closure. Their study revealed lower inspiratory volumes in individuals with upper airway closure compared to those with an open airway, with more pronounced changes at higher pressures.[19] The inspiratory volume indicates the amount of air entering the patient's lungs, with very low volumes potentially indicating laryngeal closure due to bulbar dysfunction or poor patient coordination. However, these values are easily influenced by mask leaks.[16,60,61] **Fig. 4** illustrates a titration algorithm for MI-E, including the assessment of the upper airway to achieve both efficient and tolerated treatment. In challenging patients, monitoring is invaluable to determine when benefit from MI-E is no longer present.

HYPERINFLATION THERAPIES

Assisted inflation therapies such as GPB, LVR, and mechanical inflation (using an MI-E or NIV device) are important tools in the proximal airway clearance toolbox. These techniques augment CPF,[62] and are recommended to improve cough effectiveness.[3,7,10-12,63] Some disease-specific guidelines provide thresholds for initiating therapy, (eg, assisted coughing once FVC<50% predicted, CPF<270 L/min, or MEP<60 cmH_2O[7]), whereas others advocate a more person-centered approach, "based on local resources, expertise, and shared decision-making with patients."[3]

Evidence of a physiologic effect on lung volumes is less clear. Whilst improvement in FVC has been demonstrated in children and young adults with NMDs immediately following a single session of LVR or MI-E,[28,30] other research suggests hyperinflation does not increase lung volumes or expiratory flow,[24,27,29,33,64] presumably due to participants having more severe ventilatory restriction or longer standing disease that is less amenable to change. Similarly, there is no clear

evidence that hyperinflation therapy uniformly improves ventilation distribution, airway resistance, or lung periphery reactance in the absence of an acute respiratory infection.[23-26] Variability amongst participants is seen, however,[25] and it may be that a more individualized approach is required to optimize therapies to see short-term benefits.

Looking beyond pure "airway clearance," clinical rationale and expert opinion are that routine LVR may prevent chest wall stiffness, potentially slow the decline in lung capacity, and reduce pulmonary morbidity.[3,7] However, level 1 evidence is lacking. Two randomized controlled trials (RCTs) examining the effects of twice-daily hyperinflation in children and young adults with congenital muscular dystrophies failed to show a significant benefit on the rate of FVC decline following 1[32] or 2[31] years of therapy. A shorter RCT in adults demonstrated an improvement in the volume of air inflated (lung insufflation capacity) following 3 months of twice-daily LVR, but no effect on lung volumes or respiratory system compliance.[33] Whilst these studies could be interpreted as providing little evidence for regular hyperinflation therapies, it is important to acknowledge their limitations. Average age in the pediatric studies was around 10 to 11 years,[31,32] and DMD participants had normal to very mild ventilatory restriction,[31] which may be too early in disease evolution for chest wall stiffness to present. Ventilation use was not reported by Sawnani and colleagues[32] and may confound a treatment effect. The adult trial[33] comprised people with moderately severe to severe restriction. However in this mature population, hyperinflation therapy may have been commenced too late or not performed for a long enough period to demonstrate a change in

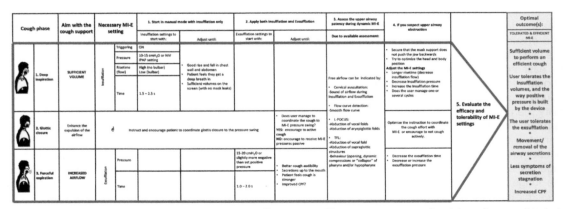

Fig. 4. Titration algorithm for mechanical insufflation-exsufflation. Titration algorithm for mechanical insufflation-exsufflation (MI-E) settings including the assessment of the upper airway to achieve both efficient and tolerated treatment. CPF, cough peak flow; IPAP, inspiratory positive airway pressure; L-POCUS, laryngeal point of care ultrasound; NIV, noninvasive ventilation; TFL, transnasal fiberoptic laryngoscopy.

respiratory system mechanics.[33] Notably, all three trials reported objectively measured adherence rates of approximately 40%,[31–33] highlighting the challenge of incorporating regular exercise into routines, even in well-supported research trial environments.

These three RCTs provide important findings to guide the clinical use of regular LVR. They illustrate the nuanced approach that is needed when prescribing a daily exercise, particularly in pwNMD. Commencing too early when there are few perceived symptoms may contribute to individuals devaluing and disregarding the therapy, whereas commencing too late may be futile. Qualitative interviews of the DMD RCT sample confirm these themes.[65] Competing activities, time burden, absence of daily sputum load, and lack of immediate perceived benefits have been implicated in low usage.[32,54] Parents and children were more motivated to use LVR following respiratory illness, and less likely during periods of stability. Conversely, despite being an easy technique to use, some families reported needing time to acclimatize and feel confident to ensure familiarity is gained before a respiratory exacerbation.[65] These findings indicate that an individualized approach to introducing LVR is needed (**Fig. 5** for a suggested algorithm). Decision-making should also take into account the emotional impact. Some families view LVR as a positive therapy that offers long-term hope, whereas others view it as a sign of disease progression, and a treatment burden.[65] A

UK-based expert respiratory working group recently published consensus recommendations for DMD care, advocating using threshold values of CPF and VC to trigger referral to specialist respiratory services where therapies can be considered and an appropriate management plan formed with patients and carers.[66]

PERIPHERAL AIRWAY CLEARANCE TECHNIQUES

With improved survival and changes in natural history, more pwNMD are presenting with issues of secretion retention. PwNMD may present with longer MI-E treatment times or chronic bacterial colonization. Bronchiectasis is common in all pediatric SMA types, with a prevalence of 1 in 5 children.[67] *Pseudomonas aeruginosa* (PSA) (38%) and *Staphylococcus aureus* (19.6%) have been identified as the most common bacteria, with a higher incidence of PSA in type I SMA.[68] Clinically, bronchiectasis and sputum retention is also seen in other NMDs where NIV has changed the natural history. Peripheral ACTs are essential in these patients. Oscillatory devices like high-flow chest oscillation or compression, and IPV have been shown to decrease hospitalizations and requirement for antibiotics.[69–71] Expiratory flow acceleration (EFA) is a technique that increases expiratory flow and enhances natural secretion movement via vacuum technology. EFA has been shown to be effective in decreasing hospitalizations and

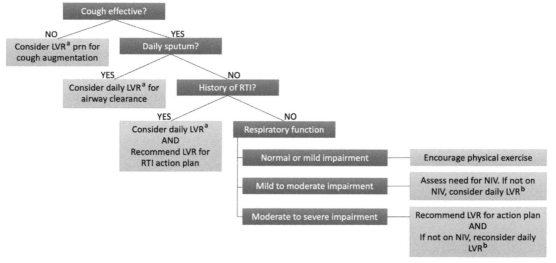

Fig. 5. Clinical algorithm to guide LVR initiation in pwNMD. Suggested clinical decision-making tree to help guide initiation of LVR in pwNMD. Consideration must include the person's goals of therapy and balance potential benefits of hyperinflation therapy with potential risks (including burden, emotional impact, pneumothorax, and other side effects). A trial of LVR may also be warranted if mechanical insufflation-exsufflation (MI-E) is indicated and not available (eg, due to cost, access). LVR, lung volume recruitment; RTI, respiratory tract infection. [a]or other ACT, [b]or other hyperinflation technique.

antibiotic requirement with pwNMD and cerebral palsy.[72,73] When EFA was used in addition to MI-E in patients with ALS, no benefit was seen with regard to hospitalizations, although the decline in lung function was slower.[60] These techniques can be used in the acute and long-term setting to mobilize secretions from the peripheral airways toward the central airways. As in other diseases,[74] no one technique has been shown to be more effective in pwNMD, and treatment should be individualized to the pwNMD and the local availability of techniques and expertize. A suggested clinical algorithm for peripheral ACT in pwNMD is shown in **Fig. 6**.

In addition to peripheral ACTs in pwNMD, there continues to be no evidence base around mucolytics in pwNMD. One recent small study has shown nebulized saline or hypertonic saline to be effective in decreasing hospitalizations in pwNMD.[75]

CHALLENGES
Treatment Adherence

Many factors influence ACT adherence in pwNMD. Long-term MI-E usage data illustrate great heterogeneity, with some users performing MI-E several times daily and some never.[22,76] Children may use MI-E more frequently than adults,[22,54,77] perhaps attributable to their young age, cognitive limitations affecting treatment options, and age-related treatment goals (ie, hyperinflation with MI-E to prevent chest wall deformity in infants with NMDs).[22,54,77,78] Hov and coworkers[22]

revealed that 74% of children using MI-E employed the treatment for both the prevention and treatment of RTIs, while 21% used it solely in the presence of excessive airway secretions. Those using MI-E treatment more frequently also place more value on it, potentially reflecting a relationship between necessity and severity.[22,54]

User and caregiver training has also been shown to affect treatment adherence.[76,79] Insufficient education, lack of follow-up, and inadequate awareness among non-specialist health care providers were identified as barriers to MI-E adherence, whereas effective initial training, caregiver support, the device's ease of use, and symptom relief facilitated MI-E usage.[79]

Equipment Access

The range of devices utilized for airway clearance and respiratory care of pwNMD is illustrated in **Fig. 1**. Whilst some of these are inexpensive, many others cost thousands of dollars or euros. Availability and cost of devices, particularly in low-income and middle-income countries, have been highlighted as barriers to implementation of international guidelines.[11,12,80] Funding models for supplying home devices vary globally and access to equipment is not equitable, even within local contexts.[34]

Professional Education

There is considerable variation in clinical education and training globally around clinical care of

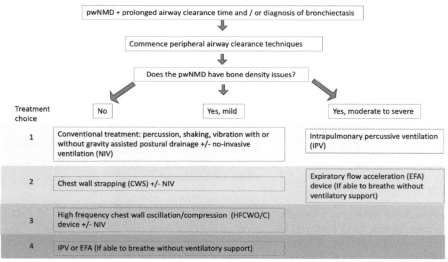

Fig. 6. Clinical algorithm for peripheral airway clearance techniques (ACTs) in people with neuromuscular disease (pwNMD). Suggested clinical algorithm for pwNMD who have prolonged issues in clearing secretions with mechanical insufflation-exsufflation (MI-E) or have had a diagnosis of chronic suppurative lung disease. This algorithm has been generated taking into account the cost of the techniques along with the availability. It also takes into account the limited evidence base in this area.

pwNMD, impacting the consistent implementation of ACTs. Low confidence, inadequate training, and limited experience and knowledge of MI-E among health care providers have been shown to pose barriers to long-term MI-E use.[79,81,82] Online, self-directed learning is an effective method for training.[83] Similarly, massive open online courses have been used to upskill large numbers of clinicians remotely. These share similarities with online e-learning modules (eg, reviewing online lectures and self-directed reading material, working through case studies and self-assessment tasks), but differ in that they have an online forum that provides participants with opportunities to engage with fellow students and teachers.[84] Whilst online learning cannot replicate face-to-face practical training sessions, remote multimodal learning models provide an alternative model of education that may address some of the barriers to training health professionals in the specialized area of respiratory management in pwNMD.

SUMMARY

Airway clearance and other respiratory therapies are a key component of the holistic management of many pwNMD. Respiratory muscle weakness leads to hypoventilation, sleep-disordered breathing, and chronic hypercapnic respiratory failure, as well as impairment in lung capacity, cough, and ability to clear secretions. The respiratory management of pwNMD can be complex and requires a well-integrated, person-centered, multidisciplinary approach. Clinicians require well-developed critical thinking, decision-making, broad and specific knowledge and skills to comprehensively assess and manage pwNMD, recognizing physical, psychological, social, and environmental factors. There are many respiratory physiotherapy interventions available to recruit lung volume, mobilize secretions, and enhance cough—the challenge is to select and individualize the appropriate technique(s) to ensure the individual's goals are being effectively targeted, especially as their disease progresses.

Recommendations

- Regular assessment of the clinical indication and effectiveness of ACTs and other respiratory therapies is needed when caring for pwNMD. Frequency of re-evaluation will be influenced by the person's symptoms, rate of disease progression, and other multidisciplinary care needs.
- Clinicians are advised to assess and consider upper airway responses during titration of MI-E more thoroughly.

- LVR might be beneficial for certain individuals but should be approached in a personalized manner.
- For individuals experiencing prolonged challenges in clearing secretions with MI-E or those diagnosed with chronic suppurative lung disease, it is recommended to consider additional peripheral ACTs.
- The holistic approach should further consider the cost and availability of techniques and the limited evidence base in this particular domain.

DISCLOSURES

N. L. Sheers is supported by a Motor Neurone Disease Research Australia (MNDRA) Jim Zissimopoulos MND Postdoctoral Fellowship (2024-2026). MNDRA has played no role in this work. T. Andersen is supported by a Western Norway Health Authorities Postdoctoral Scholarship. The funder has played no role in this work. M. Chatwin discloses she works in a noncommercial role for Breas Medical as Head of Education and Research 3 days a week. The article was carried out in her own time and Breas Medical has had no input into it.

REFERENCES

1. Poponick JM, Jacobs I, Supinski G, et al. Effect of upper respiratory tract infection in patients with neuromuscular disease. Am J Respir Crit Care Med 1997;156(2 Pt 1):659–64.
2. O'Brien D, Stavroulakis T, Baxter S, et al. The optimisation of noninvasive ventilation in amyotrophic lateral sclerosis: a systematic review. Eur Respir J 2019;54(3):1900261.
3. Khan A, Frazer-Green L, Amin R, et al. Respiratory management of patients with neuromuscular weakness: an American College of Chest Physicians clinical practice guideline and expert panel report. Chest 2023.
4. Annane D, Orlikowski D, Chevret S. Nocturnal mechanical ventilation for chronic hypoventilation in patients with neuromuscular and chest wall disorders. Cochrane Database Syst Rev 2014;(12).
5. Miller RG, Jackson CE, Kasarskis EJ, et al. Practice parameter update: the care of the patient with amyotrophic lateral sclerosis: drug, nutritional, and respiratory therapies (an evidence-based review): report of the Quality Standards Subcommittee of the American Academy of Neurology. Neurology 2009;73(15):1218–26.
6. Finkel RS, Mercuri E, Meyer OH, et al. Diagnosis and management of spinal muscular atrophy: Part 2: pulmonary and acute care; medications, supplements

and immunizations; other organ systems; and ethics. Neuromuscul Disord 2018;28(3):197–207.

7. Birnkrant DJ, Bushby K, Bann CM, et al. Diagnosis and management of Duchenne muscular dystrophy, part 2: respiratory, cardiac, bone health, and orthopaedic management. Lancet Neurol 2018;17(4): 347–61.

8. McKim DA, Road J, Avendano M, et al. Home mechanical ventilation: a Canadian Thoracic Society clinical practice guideline. Cancer Res J 2011; 18(4):197–215.

9. National Institute for Health and Clinical Excellence, NICE guideline NG42: motor neurone disease: assessment and management, Available at: https:// www.nice.org.uk/guidance/ng42, 2016. Accessed April 3, 2024.

10. Georges M, Perez T, Rabec C, et al. Proposals from a French expert panel for respiratory care in ALS patients. Respir Med Res 2022;81.

11. Toussaint M, Chatwin M, Gonzales J, et al, The ENMC Respiratory Therapy Consortium. 228th ENMC International Workshop: zirway clearance techniques in neuromuscular disorders; Naarden, The Netherlands, 3-5 March, 2017. Neuromuscul Disord 2018;28(3):289–98.

12. Chatwin M, Toussaint M, Gonçalves MR, et al. Airway clearance techniques in neuromuscular disorders: a state of the art review. Respir Med 2018; 136:98–110.

13. Sheers N, Howard ME, Berlowitz DJ. Respiratory adjuncts to NIV in neuromuscular disease. Respirology 2019;24(6):512–20.

14. Lannefors L, Button BM, McIlwaine M. Physiotherapy in infants and young children with cystic fibrosis: current practice and future developments. J R Soc Med 2004;97(44):8–25.

15. Andersen TM, Vollsæter M. Go with the flow: are we cracking the code? Respiratory management of bulbar ALS is evolving. Respir Care 2022;67(10): 1363–5.

16. Andersen TM, Fondenes O, Røksund OD, et al. From bedside to bench - in vivo and in vitro evaluation of mechanically assisted cough treatment in a patient with bulbar amyotrophic lateral sclerosis. Respir Med Case Rep 2022;37.

17. Andersen TM, Hov B, Halvorsen T, et al. Upper airway assessment and responses during mechanically assisted cough. Respir Care 2021;66(7): 1196–213.

18. Andersen TM, Sandnes A, Fondenes O, et al. Laryngeal responses to mechanically assisted cough in progressing amyotrophic lateral sclerosis. Respir Care 2018;63(5):538–49.

19. Sancho J, Ferrer S, Bures E, et al. Waveforms analysis in patients with amyotrophic lateral sclerosis for enhanced efficacy of mechanically assisted coughing. Respir Care 2022;67(10):1226–35.

20. Hov B, Andersen T, Hovland V, et al. The clinical use of mechanical insufflation-exsufflation in children with neuromuscular disorders in Europe. Paediatr Respir Rev 2018. https://doi.org/10.1016/j.prrv.2017.08.003.

21. Hov B, Carlsen KCL, Hovland V, et al. Optimizing expiratory flows during mechanical cough in a pediatric neuromuscular lung model. Pediatr Pulmonol 2020;55(2):433–40.

22. Hov B, Hovland V, Andersen T, et al. Prevalence of long-term mechanical insufflation-exsufflation in children with neurological conditions: a population-based study. Dev Med Child Neurol 2021;63(5): 537–44.

23. Steindor M, Pichler A, Heitschmidt L, et al. Multiple breath washout lung function reveals ventilation inhomogeneity unresponsive to mechanical assisted cough in patients with neuromuscular disease. BMC Pulm Med 2022;22(1):217.

24. Casaulta C, Messerli F, Rodriguez R, et al. Changes in ventilation distribution in children with neuromuscular disease using the insufflator/exsufflator technique: an observational study. Sci Rep 2022;12(1): 7009.

25. Pigatto AV, Kao TJ, Mueller JL, et al. Electrical impedance tomography detects changes in ventilation after airway clearance in spinal muscular atrophy type I. Respir Physiol Neurobiol 2021;294: 103773.

26. Pellegrino GM, Corbo M, Marco FD, et al. Effects of air stacking on dyspnea and lung function in neuromuscular diseases. Arch Phys Med Rehabil 2021; 102(8):1562–7.

27. Sheers NL, Berlowitz DJ, Dirago RK, et al. Rapidly and slowly progressive neuromuscular disease: differences in pulmonary function, respiratory tract infections and response to lung volume recruitment therapy (LVR). BMJ Open Respir Res 2022;9(1).

28. Veldhoen ES, Vercoelen F, Ros L, et al. Short-term effect of air stacking and mechanical insufflation-exsufflation on lung function in patients with neuromuscular diseases. Chron Respir Dis 2022;19. 14799731221094619.

29. Cesareo A, LoMauro A, Santi M, et al. Acute effects of mechanical insufflation-exsufflation on the breathing pattern in stable subjects with Duchenne muscular dystrophy. Respir Care 2018;63(8): 955–65.

30. Meric H, Falaize L, Pradon D, et al. Short-term effect of volume recruitment–derecruitment manoeuvre on chest-wall motion in Duchenne muscular dystrophy. Chron Respir Dis 2017;14(2):110–6.

31. Katz SL, Mah JK, McMillan HJ, et al. Routine lung volume recruitment in boys with Duchenne muscular dystrophy: a randomised clinical trial. Thorax 2022; 77(8):805–11.

32. Sawnani H, Mayer OH, Modi AC, et al. Randomized trial of lung hyperinflation therapy in children with

congenital muscular dystrophy. Pediatr Pulmonol 2020;55(9):2471–8.

33. Sheers NL, Howard ME, Rochford PD, et al. A randomised controlled trial of lung volume recruitment in adults with neuromuscular disease. Ann Am Thorac Soc 2023;20(10):1445–55.

34. Berlowitz DJ, Mathers S, Hutchinson K, et al. The complexity of multidisciplinary respiratory care in amyotrophic lateral sclerosis. Breathe 2023;19(3):220269.

35. Tabor-Gray L, Vasilopoulos T, Plowman EK. Differences in voluntary and reflexive cough strength in individuals with amyotrophic lateral sclerosis and healthy adults. Muscle Nerve 2020;62(5):597–600.

36. Rose L, McKim D, Leasa D, et al. Monitoring cough effectiveness and use of airway clearance strategies: a Canadian and UK survey. Respir Care 2018;63(12):1506–13.

37. Sancho J, Servera E, Bañuls P, et al. Effectiveness of assisted and unassisted cough capacity in amyotrophic lateral sclerosis patients. Amyotroph Lateral Scler Frontotemporal Degener 2017;18(7–8):498–504.

38. Borders JC, Brandimore AE, Troche MS. Variability of voluntary cough airflow in healthy adults and Parkinson's disease. Dysphagia 2021;36(4):700–6.

39. Laciuga H, Brandimore AE, Troche MS, et al. Analysis of clinicians' perceptual cough evaluation. Dysphagia 2016;31(4):521–30.

40. Sancho J, Servera E, Diaz J, et al. Predictors of ineffective cough during a chest infection in patients with stable amyotrophic lateral sclerosis. Am J Respir Crit Care Med 2007;175(12):1266–71.

41. Lacombe M, Boré A, Amo Castrillo LD, et al. Peak cough flow fails to detect upper airway collapse during negative pressure titration for Cough-Assist. Arch Phys Med Rehabil 2019;100(12):2346–53.

42. Ren S, Cai M, Shi Y, et al. Influence of cough airflow characteristics on respiratory mucus clearance. Phys Fluids 2022;34(4):041911.

43. Brandimore AE, Troche MS, Huber JE, et al. Respiratory kinematic and airflow differences between reflex and voluntary cough in healthy young adults. Front Physiol 2015;6.

44. Szeinberg A, Tabachnik E, Rashed N, et al. Cough capacity in patients with muscular dystrophy. Chest 1988;94(6):1232–5.

45. Umayahara Y, Soh Z, Sekikawa K, et al. Estimation of cough peak flow using cough sounds. Sensors 2018;18:2381.

46. Recasens BB, Balana Corbero A, Llorens JMM, et al. Sound-based cough peak flow estimation in patients with neuromuscular disorders. Muscle Nerve 2024;69(2):213–7.

47. Chatwin M, Wakeman RH. Mechanical insufflation-exsufflation: considerations for improving clinical practice. J Clin Med 2023;12(7):2626.

48. Troxell DA, Bach JR, Nilsestuen JO. Mechanical insufflation-exsufflation implementation and management, aided by graphics analysis. Chest 2023;164(6):1505–11.

49. Lalmolda C, Prados H, Mateu G, et al. Titration of mechanical insufflation–exsufflation optimal pressure combinations in neuromuscular diseases by flow/pressure waveform analysis. Arch Bronconeumol 2019;55(5):246–51.

50. Bianchi C, Baiardi P. Cough peak flows: standard values for children and adolescents. Am J Phys Med Rehabil 2008;87(6):461–7.

51. Toussaint M, Boitano LJ, Gathot V, et al. Limits of effective cough-augmentation techniques in patients with neuromuscular disease. Respir Care 2009;54(3):359–66.

52. Kotwal N, Shukla PJ, Perez GF. Peak cough flow in children with neuromuscular disorders. Lung 2020;198(2):371–5.

53. LoMauro A, Romei M, D'Angelo MG, et al. Determinants of cough efficiency in Duchenne muscular dystrophy. Pediatr Pulmonol 2014;49(4):357–65.

54. Chatwin M, Simonds AK. Long-term mechanical insufflation-exsufflation cough assistance in neuromuscular disease: patterns of use and lessons for application. Respir Care 2020;65(2):135.

55. Hov B, Andersen T, Toussaint M, et al. Mechanically assisted cough strategies: user perspectives and cough flows in children with neurodisability. ERJ Open Res 2024;10.

56. Andersen T, Sandnes A, Brekka AK, et al. Laryngeal response patterns influence the efficacy of mechanical assisted cough in amyotrophic lateral sclerosis. Thorax 2017;72(3):221.

57. Andersen T, Sandnes A, Hilland M, et al. Laryngeal response patterns to mechanical insufflation-exsufflation in healthy subjects 2013;92(10):920–9.

58. Vollsaeter M, Skjoldmo A, Røksund O, et al. Tailoring NIV by dynamic laryngoscopy in a child with spinal muscular atrophy type I. Clin Case Rep 2021;9:1925–8.

59. Marrara JL, Duca AP, Dantas RO, et al. Swallowing in children with neurologic disorders: clinical and videofluoroscopic evaluations. Pro Fono 2008;20(4):231–6.

60. Nicolini A, Prato P, Beccarelli L, et al. Comparison of two mechanical insufflation-exsufflation devices in patients with amyotrophic lateral sclerosis: a preliminary study. Panminerva Med 2022;64(4):525–31.

61. Gomaa D, Benditt JO, Hanseman D, et al. Comparison of mechanical insufflation-exsufflation using a stand alone device and integrated into a ventilator. Respir Care 2019;64(Suppl 10):3239521.

62. Sheers NL, O'Sullivan R, Howard ME, et al. The role of lung volume recruitment therapy in neuromuscular disease: a narrative review. Frontiers Rehab Sci 2023;4:1164628.

63. Quinlivan R, Astin R, Khan J, et al. Adult North Star Network (ANSN): consensus guideline for the standard of care of adults with Duchenne muscular dystrophy. J Neuromuscul Dis 2021;8(6):899–926.

64. Molgat-Seon Y, Hannan LM, Dominelli PB, et al. Lung volume recruitment acutely increases respiratory system compliance in individuals with severe respiratory muscle weakness. ERJ Open Res 2017; 3(1):00135–2016.

65. Katz SL, Blinder H, Newhook D, et al. Understanding the experiences of lung volume recruitment among boys with Duchenne muscular dystrophy: a multicenter qualitative study. Pediatr Pulmonol 2023; 58(1):46–54.

66. Childs AM, Turner C, Astin R, et al. Development of respiratory care guidelines for Duchenne muscular dystrophy in the UK: key recommendations for clinical practice. Thorax 2023;79(5):476–85.

67. Chacko A, Sly PD, Gauld LM, et al. Dysphagia and lung disease in children with spinal muscular atrophy treated with disease-modifying agents. Neurology 2023;100(19):914–20.

68. Levine H, Nevo Y, Katz J, et al. Evaluation of sputum cultures in children with spinal muscular atrophy. Respir Med 2023;209.

69. Yuan N, Shelton K, Matel J, et al. Safety, tolerability, and efficacy of high-frequency chest wall oscillation in pediatric patients with cerebral palsy and neuromuscular diseases: an exploratory randomized controlled trial. J Child Neurol 2010;25(7):815–21.

70. Lechtzin N, Wolfe LF, Frick KD. The impact of high-frequency chest wall oscillation on healthcare use in patients with neuromuscular diseases. Ann Am Thorac Soc 2016;13(6):904–9.

71. Bidiwala A, Volpe L, Halaby C, et al. A comparison of high frequency chest wall oscillation and intrapulmonary percussive ventilation for airway clearance in pediatric patients with tracheostomy. Postgrad Med 2017;129(2):276–82.

72. Bertelli L, Bardasi G, Di Palmo E, et al. Airway clearance management with Vaküm technology in subjects with ineffective cough: a pilot study on the efficacy, acceptability evaluation, and perception in children with cerebral palsy. Pediatr Allergy Immunol Pulmonol 2019;32(1):23–7.

73. Garuti G, Giovannini M, Verucchi E, et al. Management of bronchial secretions with Free Aspire in children with cerebral palsy: impact on clinical outcomes and healthcare resources. Ital J Pediatr 2016;42(1).

74. Main E, Rand S. Conventional chest physiotherapy compared to other airway clearance techniques for cystic fibrosis. Cochrane Database Syst Rev 2023;(5).

75. Galaz Souza N, Bush A, Tan H-L. Exploratory study of the effectiveness of nebulised saline in children with neurodisability. Eur Respir J 2021;57(3): 2001407.

76. Siewers V, Holmøy T, Frich JC. Experiences with using mechanical in-exsufflation in amyotrophic lateral sclerosis. Eur J Physiother 2013;15(4):201–7.

77. Mahede T, Davis G, Rutkay A, et al. Use of mechanical airway clearance devices in the home by people with neuromuscular disorders: effects on health service use and lifestyle benefits. Orphanet J Rare Dis 2015;10(1):1–7.

78. Chatwin M, Bush A, Simonds AK. Outcome of goal-directed non-invasive ventilation and mechanical insufflation/exsufflation in spinal muscular atrophy type I. Arch Dis Child 2011;96(5):426–32.

79. Dale CM, McKim D, Amin R, et al. Education experiences of adult subjects and caregivers for mechanical insufflation-exsufflation at home. Respir Care 2020;65(12):1889–96.

80. Human A, Corten L, Morrow BM. The role of physiotherapy in the respiratory management of children with neuromuscular diseases: a South African perspective. S Afr J Physiother 2021;77(1):1–11.

81. Rose L, Adhikari NK, Poon J, et al. Cough augmentation techniques in the critically ill: a Canadian national survey. Respir Care 2016;61(10):1360–8.

82. Swingwood EL, Stilma W, Tume LN, et al. The use of mechanical insufflation-exsufflation in invasively ventilated critically ill adults. Respir Care 2022; 67(8):1043–57.

83. Lambrinos E, Elkins MR, Menadue C, et al. Online education improves confidence in mechanical insufflation-exsufflation. Respir Care 2023;69(1):91–8.

84. Harvey LA, Glinsky JV, Lowe R, et al. A Massive Open Online Course for teaching physiotherapy students and physiotherapists about spinal cord injuries. Spinal Cord 2014;52(12):911–8.

Palliative Care and Noninvasive Ventilation

Tracy A. Smith, BSc, MBBS, PhD[a,b,*], Mary M. Roberts, MSN, BHS, MSPC, DipAppSc(nursing)[a,b,c,d], Lesley Howard, BAppSc, MHlthSc[a]

KEYWORDS

- Advance care planning (ACP) • Chronic obstructive pulmonary disease (COPD) • End-of-life care
- Neuromuscular disease • Noninvasive ventilation (NIV) • Palliative care

KEY POINTS

- Timely introduction of palliative care is important in patients treated with noninvasive ventilation (NIV). Difficulties with prognostication in this patient group should not be a barrier to proactive discussion of symptom relief and advance care planning.
- The commencement of NIV is often an appropriate trigger to discuss advance care planning and introduce palliative care.
- Weaning NIV at the end of life is often appropriate; however, the evidence base to guide clinicians is sparse.

PALLIATIVE CARE—DEFINITION AND RELATION TO NONINVASIVE VENTILATION

At first sight, noninvasive ventilation (NIV) and palliative care may appear diametrically opposed. NIV is used acutely in the management of respiratory failure due to a new-onset, reversible cause,[1] or in the long-term management of chronic respiratory failure.[2,3] In contrast, palliative care is often associated with the end of life. However, a broader understanding of the role of palliative care and how patients' care needs might change over time is key to appreciating the importance of the relationship.

Some patients who require NIV for slowly progressive neuromuscular diseases, for instance Duchenne muscular dystrophy, may have a good long-term outlook.[4] However, other patients requiring NIV will have a chronic cardiorespiratory disease,[3] or more rapidly progressive neuromuscular disease, like motor neurone disease (MND), which likely portends a more guarded prognosis. Some investigators have used the term "palliative NIV" to refer to patients with orders to "do not intubate," or "comfort measures only," who require NIV.[5] However, restricting discussion of palliative care in NIV only to this group misses a large patient population that has the potential to benefit from principles of care which arise from a palliative approach.

The World Health Organization's definition of palliative care encompasses assessment and management of symptoms, be they physical, emotional, or spiritual,[6] and does not specify a time frame for these in relation to the end of life. Chronic cardiorespiratory disease and neuromuscular disease are life-limiting diagnoses. NIV may be required either acutely or chronically for these patients. Between 'now' and the end of life, patients will have symptoms and other concerns.

[a] Department of Respiratory and Sleep Medicine, Westmead Hospital, Western Sydney Local Health District, New South Wales, Australia; [b] The University of Sydney, Faculty of Medicine and Health, Westmead Clinical School, New South Wales, Australia; [c] Ludwig Engel Centre for Respiratory Research, Westmead Institute for Medical Research, Westmead, New South Wales, Australia; [d] Improving Palliative Care, Aged and Chronic Care through Clinical Research and Translation (IMPACCT), University of Technology, New South Wales, Australia
* Corresponding author. Department of Respiratory and Sleep Medicine, Westmead Hospital, PO Box 533, Westmead 2145.
E-mail address: tracy.smith2@health.nsw.gov.au

Sleep Med Clin 19 (2024) 497–507
https://doi.org/10.1016/j.jsmc.2024.04.010

Addressing these aspects is key to excellent clinical care and is the essence of palliative care. Further, specific palliative care strategies may be required in the last days of life. While this is important work, it is a minority of what palliative care is about.

Fig. 1 illustrates a variety of pathways that may be followed by people with different diseases as the end of life approaches.[7] Patients requiring NIV may have a diversity of illnesses leading to the requirement for NIV. Those with neuromuscular disease and chronic obstructive pulmonary disease (COPD) will most likely follow a chronic disease–type pathway. In this trajectory, patients have periods of good health, punctuated with periods of worse health and the hope to recover to their previous level. Even though deterioration has occurred over a prolonged period for patients following this trajectory, death will often seem "sudden" to families.[8]

Prognosticating in both respiratory and neuromuscular disease is notoriously difficult, and this is often cited as a barrier to beginning discussions of palliative care or advance care planning (ACP). Rather than seeing palliative care as a "referral of last resort" to be made when "nothing else can be done," NIV clinicians should regard palliative care as an adjunct to usual care. Indeed, usual care and palliative care may exist concurrently (**Fig. 2**). When done well, discussions about symptom burden and preferences regarding disease management need to evolve over time. It's never too early to ask patients about symptoms or preferences should their health deteriorate. Health professionals should be proactive in opening these discussions as patients often wait until they are broached by their care team rather than opening discussions themselves.[9,10]

In the acute setting, NIV may offer both benefits and burdens. These are summarized in **Table 1**. The transition from acute care to end-of-life care has been identified as a key transition for people who use long-term NIV.[11] Despite both patients and clinicians recognizing the importance of this transition, it is rarely discussed.[11] The reasons for this are complex and involve questions of prognosis,

Proposed Trajectories of Dying

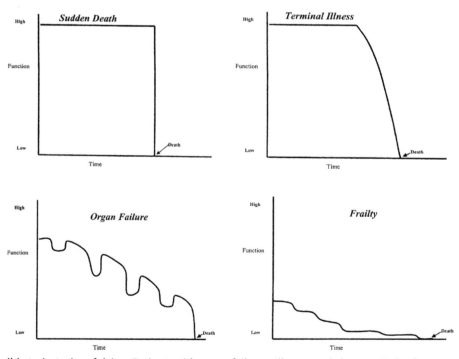

Fig. 1. Possible trajectories of dying. Patients with organ failure will commonly have periods of worsening health, often due to acute medical events. While recovery is common, it is often incomplete. Prognosticating as to whether 'this' episode of deterioration will result in recovery or death can be difficult. Patients with terminal illness (often malignancy) often have an evident period of decline, and death may be more easily predicted. (*From[7]* with permission)

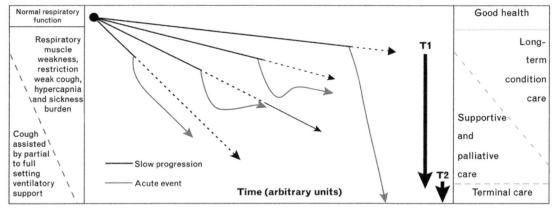

Fig. 2. Trajectories of change in progressive motor neurone disease. Solid black lines represent clinical change. Gray lines represent change accelerated by acute events (infection, aspiration, and so forth). Recovery following these deteriorations may be incomplete, and any event may progress to become a terminal deterioration. The right panel represents the integration of palliative care through illness progression. (*From*[19] with permission)

as well as the unpredictable progression of some illnesses that require NIV. Proactive discussion of ACP is recommended but often does not occur.

ADVANCE CARE PLANNING—DEFINITION AND RELATION TO NONINVASIVE VENTILATION

ACP is "a process that supports adults at any age or stage of health in understanding and sharing their personal values, life goals, and preferences regarding future medical care. The goal of ACP is to help ensure that people receive medical care that is consistent with their values, goals, and preferences during serious and chronic illness."[12]

ACP previously focused on producing an advance care directive.[13] More recent understandings suggest it is an ongoing social process that includes the patient, their family, and health care providers reflecting and discussing goals and values to inform current and future medical care.[14,15] The use of the word 'family' is inclusive of those close to the patient as well as those actually related.

ACP is recommended for all patients with chronic life-limiting illnesses.[16] International professional societies recognize that ACP is an integral duty of care that should be provided to patients with life-limiting respiratory diseases.[17,18] Similar recommendations are made for patients with neuromuscular diseases.[19] However, difficulties in prognostication may deter some clinicians. The need for NIV may portend a poor prognosis and may therefore provide a good trigger for discussion.[20–22]

ACP conversations should occur when the patient is still relatively well and can actively participate rather than during a crisis.[23] In a crisis, patients have a reduced capacity to participate in decision-making, and time for comprehensive discussions is limited. Further, key people,

Table 1
Benefits and burdens of noninvasive ventilation in the acute setting

Benefits	Burdens
Support of respiration while potentially reversible causes of respiratory failure (eg, infection, fluid overload) are treated	Added decision-making burden for patient, family, and health professionals if NIV needs to be withdrawn
May improve breathlessness and/or allow time to institute pharmacologic measures to improve breathlessness	May add to discomfort, and thereby add to suffering
May 'buy time' to allow arrival of family	May prolong the dying process
	NIV interface may be a barrier to conversation and/or prevent physical expressions of care (eg, a kiss on the cheek)

Abbreviation: NIV, noninvasive ventilation.

Box 1
Essential components of an advance care planning discussion

Assessing the patient's (and their family's) readiness to participate in such conversation

- Proactively offer to discuss ACP, preferably in the outpatient setting.
- Assess readiness for ACP discussions.
- Recognize initial conversations may be confronting, but most patients find these discussions positive, helpful and worthwhile.[14]

Explore the patient's understanding of their illness:

- Ask patients what they understand regarding the diagnosis, prognosis, and role of NIV.
- Clarify any misperceptions.
- Ask about fears and concerns.
- Honesty regarding prognosis is crucial.[26]
- Contrary to clinicians' concerns, ACP may build hope, confidence, and peace.[14]

Discussing values and goals of care

- Identify the patient's overall goals and priorities in life in the context of illness and NIV.
- Discuss burdens versus benefits of NIV.
- Inquire about the place of death and/or important cultural and spiritual practices.[27]

Identifying a surrogate decision-maker

- Patients may have clear views on who should, and should not, make decisions if they are too unwell to express their preferences.[22]
- Ask specifically who to involve
- The role of the surrogate decision-maker is to express what the patient would want, rather than their own opinions. Clearly explain this.[28]
- Involving surrogate decision-makers in ACP discussions enables congruity between the patient, surrogate, and clinician.[25] Up to one-third of surrogate decision-makers incorrectly predict patient preferences.[28]

Documenting discussion

- Document discussions to increase the likelihood of maintaining autonomy and having wishes known and respected.[25]
- Consider providing patients with their written directives and keeping these in a prominent place in the home for first responders.[29]

Revisiting

- Patients' goals may change as their condition changes. Revisiting ACP allows these changes to be recognized.

- Provide opportunities to discuss ACP with patients who previously declined discussion, but understand that some patients will continue to decline. Be gentle, curious and respectful.

Bausewein, C., Currow, D.C., & Johnson, M.J.. Recognising advanced disease, advance care planning and recognition of dying for people with COPD. In: Palliative Care in Respiratory Diseases (ERS Monograph). Sheffield, European Respiratory Society, 2016; pp 204-220. Reproduced with permission of the © ERS 2024.

including family, the family doctor, and usual care team, may be unavailable.[24] Conversations can be framed by 'hoping for the best, preparing for the worst,' and should focus on what will be done (nursing care, symptom relief, and so forth) rather than what will not occur (intubation/resuscitation).

Box 1 outlines the essential components that should be incorporated into an ACP discussion.[25]

Discussing ACP and palliative care requires a range of communication skills. It is inherently emotional and can be taxing. Evidence suggests clinicians may feel underprepared.[23] Key skills which may assist include

- Explicitly ask if the patient wants a surrogate decision-maker involved in discussions.
- Proactively elicit patient preferences.
- Pace the discussion. Look for nonverbal clues to people being overwhelmed or shutting down. Pause and reflect from time to time.
- Avoid jargon. Use simple, everyday language.
- Be comfortable with silence. Ask a question and be prepared to "wait for 8." That is, wait 8 seconds before filling the conversation gap. You'll be amazed at what comes up.
- Watch for, acknowledge, and respond to emotion. "You look upset; what is happening for you?"
- Foster realistic hope. False reassurance ultimately undermines the clinical alliance.
- Encourage questions.
- Use formal health care interpreters rather than family members when needed.
- Consider if there are cultural differences between patients and health providers. Use curiosity and kindness to underpin meaningful dialog while respecting differences.

While ACP is a broad discussion about preferences and values, resuscitation planning is usually important. A key trigger for clinicians is that if you would not intubate/ventilate the patient, ACP is warranted. Additionally, discussions are usually appropriate following a hospitalization characterized by acute or acute-on-chronic respiratory failure.

When discussing resuscitation, focus on what will be done rather than what will not. Discussing a plan for a time-limited trial of therapy involving restorative care (including NIV, antibiotics, corticosteroids, diuretics as required) offers a starting point. Then transitioning to a discussion of comfort-focused options can be helpful. Emphasize the ongoing provision of comfort-focused pharmacotherapy, nursing care, and family support. Finally, using phrases like "allow natural death" or "allow nature to take its course" to refer to the process of death can be helpful.

NEUROMUSCULAR DISEASE: NONINVASIVE VENTILATION AND PALLIATIVE CARE

Many neuromuscular diseases are associated with chronic, irreversible respiratory muscle weakness and the development of respiratory failure.[30] NIV is utilized by patients with respiratory muscle insufficiency in the pursuit of a number of subjective and objective goals including a reduction in breathlessness,[31] improvement in sleep quantity and quality,[32] improvements in gas exchange,[33] and improved quality of life (QOL).[34] In some patient groups, the initiation of NIV has also been shown to have benefits to life expectancy,[34,35] although in others, the benefits are largely focused on symptoms and QOL with little positive impact on life expectancy.[34]

Despite these advances in medical technology, most patients with neuromuscular disease will die of respiratory complications.[36] In fact, the commencement of NIV often signals the advancing nature of the disease. With this in mind, commencing discussions of ACP and the introduction of the concept and role of palliative care early in the management of patients with neuromuscular disease, particularly those with rapidly progressive neuromuscular disease such as MND, is recommended.[19,37]

Fig. 2 illustrates potential paths of decline in neuromuscular disease.[19] Importantly, it highlights that the transition between long-term care and supportive care as a continuum. Even in those with relatively mild impairment of respiratory function, an acute event can occur at any time and have significant, irreversible consequences. This highlights the need for early discussions of patient wishes and limits of care. The right-hand panel illustrates the overlap between long-term restorative care and palliative care. This overlap also applies to chronic cardiorespiratory disease. Given that the focus of this article is NIV, the authors have not addressed the role of cough assist

devices as mentioned in the left-hand panel but acknowledge their importance.[19]

Disease progression often leads to further respiratory muscle weakness and consequent daytime hypoventilation, breathlessness, and fatigue. Patients may begin to use NIV during waking hours either due to a recommendation from the medical team or self-initiated by the patient,[38] with some patients progressing to use NIV continuously.

Guidelines developed for the MND population have recommended that at or before the commencement of NIV, the patient and their family should receive education on the role of NIV, identifying its inherent supportive rather than curative purpose, and that the patient may elect to cease NIV at any time. ACP should include the likelihood of withdrawing NIV at the end of life. Although patients, families, and clinicians identify the withdrawal of assisted ventilation at the end of life to be a challenging concept to discuss,[39] it is recommended that this discussion begins early and be ongoing, to allow time for discussion and reflection by the patient and family.[37] Clear communication, led by an experienced clinician, and involving the patient, family, and care providers about the goals and plan for assisted ventilation throughout the dying process is key to achieving sensitive, safe, and effective palliative care.[37] This discussion is important, as while some patients will die on NIV, many will cease NIV prior to death, often in the last days of life.

CHRONIC OBSTRUCTIVE PULMONARY DISEASE: NONINVASIVE VENTILATION AND PALLIATIVE CARE

NIV is used chronically in advanced COPD with hypercapnic respiratory failure where it improves blood gas parameters, and may improve QOL with a limited impact on survival.[40] Such patients have a symptom burden often greater than patients with lung cancer, but receive less formal palliative care input.[41] The reasons for this are complex, and it has been suggested that earlier involvement of palliative care might reduce inappropriate health resource utilization as death approaches, benefitting both patients and overstretched health systems,[41–43] though a recent feasibility study of a palliative care intervention struggled to enroll patients with COPD, casting doubt on this assertion.[44]

The utility of NIV to relieve breathlessness in the chronic setting is unclear. A systematic review found a very small improvement in breathlessness as a result of chronic NIV usage, along with marginal improvements in QOL.[40] That said, qualitative[45] and questionnaire-based studies suggest improvements in breathlessness.[46] On the other hand, NIV initiation may be frightening and difficult.

Many patients with COPD will die in the acute setting, often with a trial of respiratory support. There is evidence of increasing use of NIV as the end of life approaches.[47] It is unclear if NIV relieves breathlessness toward the end of life. An older systematic review found there was insufficient data to determine in the randomized controlled trials (RCTs) of NIV for acute respiratory failure relieved breathlessness.[48] However, qualitative studies in this patient group are clear that patients report improvement in breathlessness with the initiation of NIV,[49] albeit that NIV is associated with a range of other difficult experiences and a high symptom burden.[50] An excellent review article has comprehensively explored the broader role of palliative care in COPD and is highly recommended.[51]

The need for chronic long-term NIV in COPD may be seen as a sentinel event, signifying progressive respiratory failure due to advancing disease.[52] As in neuromuscular disease, frank and open discussions regarding prognosis, the expected benefits and burdens of NIV, and palliative care should be undertaken. Additionally, parameters and preferences regarding cessation of NIV should be discussed when long-term NIV is initiated.

HIGH-FLOW NASAL PRONGS AS AN ALTERNATIVE TO NONINVASIVE VENTILATION

Recently there has been interest in the use of high-flow nasal prongs (HFNPs) in both acute and chronic settings where NIV might otherwise be used.[53,54] The advantage of HFNPs is that this technology is widely regarded as more comfortable, and facilitates easier conversation with the family, two factors which are particularly important from a palliative care point of view. One small retrospective trial from Denmark suggested HFNPs were better tolerated, especially toward the end-of-life.[55] In the setting of chronic respiratory failure, HFNPs appear to reduce hospitalizations and improve QOL compared to long-term oxygen therapy/usual care, though the impact on mortality is unclear.[53,54] The question of whether HFNPs in either the acute or chronic setting reduce important symptoms, like breathlessness, is not yet clear, and future trials should include this end point. As discussed earlier, there has been some recent work in the use of HFNPs instead of NIV in the acute setting[54] but much more work is needed here. Additionally, HFNP support has been used to facilitate death at home, which may be very important for some patients.[56]

BREATHLESSNESS MANAGEMENT

Given the predominance of this symptom in patients requiring NIV, and the importance of symptom relief in palliative care, a brief mention of measures to address this symptom is appropriate. In general, non-pharmacologic interventions can be useful in both acute breathlessness 'crises' and to reduce breathlessness during daily activities. Effective strategies include

- Use of a battery-operated hand-held fan[57]
- Pursed lip breathing — this reduces hyperinflation.
- 'Breathing around the rectangle'—long slow breath out, short breath in, long slow breath out, and so forth. This reduces hyperinflation.
- Use of a 4-wheel walker to mobilize/shower chairs to shower/terry toweling bathrobe to dry after showering

Additionally, many patients strongly believe that they will die in the middle of a breathlessness crisis. This is, however, rare in clinical practice. Providing this reassurance can be enormously comforting to the patient and their family.

Pharmacologic interventions for breathlessness can be considered but have limited efficacy. While opioids are effective for breathlessness at rest,[58] a recent study has suggested they do not assist breathlessness on exertion.[59] Benzodiazepines do not relieve breathlessness, are associated with harm, and should not be used.[60] There is limited evidence that mirtazapine may assist and an RCT for this agent is underway.[61] Other symptoms that are often prominent include dry mouth, fatigue, pain, anxiety, and depression. These should be addressed using evidence-based guidelines.

Many patients and some clinicians feel that the provision of long-term oxygen may relieve symptoms in people with advanced COPD. Oxygen improves survival and hypoxemia, and may assist with exercise-induced breathlessness, but does not improve breathlessness in daily life.[62]

WEANING NONINVASIVE VENTILATION AT THE END OF LIFE

The decision of whether to continue or cease ventilation toward the end of life is unique for each patient and their clinical situation. In the acute setting, a time-limited trial of respiratory support is often appropriate, with re-evaluation of response to treatment and patient preferences. These conversations can be difficult, and at times, clinicians may need the support of social work, pastoral care, and palliative care colleagues. In the chronic setting, patients should be made aware that it is their right to choose to discontinue treatment, and it is the duty of the medical services to support their decision and provide appropriate support to the patient and family in managing the physical and emotional consequences of this decision.[37] These discussions between the patient, family, and clinicians should be undertaken well ahead of the planned withdrawal.[37] Before ceasing ventilation, discussions with the patient and family should be undertaken including when, where, and how NIV withdrawal will occur,[37] along with providing information on what to expect once NIV is ceased.

The literature on the topic of withdrawing assisted ventilation in patients with chronic respiratory failure at the end of life is limited and, where available, is largely drawn from the MND population.[37,63] The Assocoiation for Pallitive Medicine for Great Britan and Ireland have published an excellent clinical guideline reviewing ventilation withdrawal in people with MND.[37] This outlines the options for care depending on the level of ventilator dependence, emphasizing proactive, individualized, titrated medication delivery.[37] A prospective study implementing these guidelines in an MND population found good symptom management at the end of life.[64] Most families of the deceased in this study reported that their experience of care was positive. Work available only as a conference abstract reports significantly less agitation in a mixed patient population at the time of death following institution of a framework using these principles.[65]

End-of-life care for people requiring NIV, even those who are very dependent, can be successfully managed in a variety of environments including community, hospital, or hospice.[63,64,66] The location of care will depend on patient and family preferences, as well as clinical circumstances. A dignified, comfortable death can be expected regardless of the location of care with careful planning and management.[64] Transition from NIV to HFNPs may have a role in some clinical circumstances; however, this evidence base requires development.

In circumstances where the patient or family express their preference not to cease NIV prior to death due to symptoms or concerns of hastening death, it is possible to achieve a dignified and comfortable death with NIV in place, although the option of removing NIV prior to death may be able to be revisited. Again, it is important that family members understand that their role is to represent the patient's wishes, even when they are different from their own. Attention should be paid to spiritual care for patients and families as the end of life approaches. The use of pastoral care and/or clergy is advocated when appropriate.

More research is required to better elucidate weaning protocols. Additionally, studies evaluating the quality of death and dying for patients who succumb to illness are urgently required.

Some practical points the authors have found helpful when weaning or ceasing NIV in the authors' clinical experience are outlined below.

- Consider review of ventilator settings to better align with goals of care, for example, reducing the pressures and/or backup rate in patients where symptom control can be maintained at lower settings.
- Cease monitoring of arterial blood gases.
- Review alarm settings on the ventilator and any monitoring devices.
- Where appropriate, transition to monitoring for comfort rather than assessing vital signs (where unable to transition, consider, if possible, for in-room monitoring to not display parameters or alarms).
- When the patient's level of consciousness is sufficiently reduced and/or appropriate pharmaceutical support is in progress, revisit plans for removing NIV.
- Prepare the family and staff for what to expect when a patient dies with NIV still in progress. For example, in any mode of NIV where a respiratory rate or backup rate is used, the patient may appear to continue to be breathing after they have died. Alternate means of patient assessment are required from the usual observation of chest movement. Some family members, and even some health professionals, may wrongly assume that at the time of death, the machine will turn off and/or an alarm will sound. Depending on specific settings, this may not be the case.

Box 2 summarizes the key points to consider with respect to NIV and palliative care.

VOLUNTARY ASSISTED DYING AND NONINVASIVE VENTILATION

Voluntary assisted dying is legal in a variety of jurisdictions. Individual clinicians should be aware of the laws which relate to their geographic area of practice. Often, legal frameworks for voluntary assisted dying are drafted widely enough that they may include patients who require NIV, particularly those with neuromuscular disease. Even in jurisdictions where voluntary assisted dying is not permitted, patients may ask about this area. All individuals are entitled to their views about the pros and cons of this process. It is essential that all clinicians are prepared to answer questions in this regard which honor both the patients' and

> **Box 2**
> **Key points in noninvasive ventilation and palliative care**
>
> - The introduction of the concept and role of palliative care early in the management of patients requiring NIV is recommended.[19,37,51]
> - It is important that the medical team work collaboratively with the patient and their family, considering each individual's circumstances and preferences, when planning the use of assisted ventilation in the palliative process. This process should begin early and be ongoing to provide time for careful consideration and discussions between all parties.[37]
> - A plan for symptom management is required, should be proactively considered, and be in place prior to the cessation of assisted ventilation.[39,64]
> - Patients dependent on NIV may, or may not, choose to cease NIV prior to death. In either circumstance, they can be successfully managed in the home, hospice, or institutional settings with appropriate support in place.[63,64,66]
> - ACP should be initiated by clinicians early in the disease process and revisited from time to time. This allows patients to participate as active partners in the process and allows their views to evolve as their illness progresses.
> - Communication skills necessary for conducting ACP can be learned and, like all other skills in clinical care, require practice and persistence.
> - A variety of strategies, both pharmacologic and non-pharmacologic are available to address symptoms. It is never too early to ask patients about their symptoms and offer effective interventions.
> - Patients requiring NIV for neuromuscular disease and those requiring it for COPD are different but have overlapping pallitive are needs.
> - While guidelines exist for weaning NIV at the end of life in patients with neuromuscular disease, further research is needed.

the clinicians' views. Understanding local laws, and where appropriate, local referral pathways, is an essential component of modern clinical practice. Where a patient is not appropriate according to local laws, this should be managed sensitively, and consideration of exploring previously untried means to address symptoms, as well as exploration for suicidality should be considered in the appropriate clinical circumstances.

SELF-CARE FOR CLINICIANS

It is important to acknowledge that caring for these patient populations can be difficult for the professional care team. Dealing with patients and their families' emotions can be exhausting, and grief and loss at the death of patients is common. Additionally, dealing with an ethically fraught area of care can be taxing. Teams and clinicians who provide care to these patient groups should anticipate and plan for these difficulties and take active steps to care for themselves and each other.

CLINICS CARE POINTS

- Consideration of the palliative care needs of patients requiring NIV is important. Patient symptoms and concerns should be proactively elicited and addressed.

REFERENCES

1. Rochwerg B, Brochard L, Elliott MW, et al. Official ERS/ATS clinical practice guidelines: noninvasive ventilation for acute respiratory failure. Eur Respir J 2017;50(2):1602426.
2. Khan A, Frazer-Green L, Amin R, et al. Respiratory management of patients with neuromuscular weakness: an American College of chest physicians clinical practice guideline and Expert panel report. Chest 2023;164(2):394–413.
3. Ergan B, Oczkowski S, Rochwerg B, et al. European Respiratory Society guidelines on long-term home non-invasive ventilation for management of COPD. Eur Respir J 2019;54(3):1901003.
4. Ishikawa Y, Miura T, Ishikawa Y, et al. Duchenne muscular dystrophy: survival by cardio-respiratory interventions. Neuromuscul Disord 2011;21(1):47–51.
5. Azoulay É, Demoule A, Jaber S, et al. Palliative noninvasive ventilation in patients with acute respiratory failure. Intensive Care Med 2011;37(8):1250–7.
6. World health Organization. Available at: https://www.who.int/news-room/fact-sheets/detail/palliative-care. [Accessed 6 November 2023].
7. Lunney JR, Lynn J, Hogan C. Profiles of older Medicare Decedents. J Am Geriatr Soc 2002;50(6):1108–12.
8. Murray SA, Sheikh A. Palliative care beyond cancer: care for all at the end of life. BMJ 2008;336(7650):958–9.
9. Poveda-Moral S, Falcó-Pegueroles A, Ballesteros-Silva MP, et al. Barriers to advance care planning Implementation in health care: an Umbrella review with Implications for evidence-based practice.

Worldviews Evidence-Based Nurs 2021;18(5): 254–63.

10. Johnson S, Butow P, Kerridge I, et al. Advance care planning for cancer patients: a systematic review of perceptions and experiences of patients, families, and healthcare providers. Psycho Oncol 2016; 25(4):362–86.

11. Xiao L, Amin R, Nonoyama ML. Long-term mechanical ventilation and transitions in care: a narrative review. Chron Respir Dis 2023;20:1–12.

12. Sudore RLMD, Lum HD, You JJ, et al. Defining advance care planning for adults: a Consensus definition from a Multidisciplinary Delphi panel. J Pain Symptom Manag 2017;53(5):821–32.e1.

13. Brinkman-Stoppelenburg A, Rietjens JAC, van der Heide A. The effects of advance care planning on end-of-life care: a systematic review. Palliat Med 2014;28(8):1000–25.

14. Hall A, Rowland C, Grande G. How should end-of-life advance care planning discussions Be implemented according to patients and informal Carers? A qualitative review of reviews. J Pain Symptom Manag 2019;58(2):311–35.

15. Jimenez G, Tan WS, Virk AK, et al. Overview of systematic reviews of advance care planning: Summary of evidence and Global Lessons. J Pain Symptom Manag 2018;56(3):436–59.e25.

16. Gallagher R. An approach to advance care planning in the office. Can Fam Physician 2006;52(4):459–64.

17. Andreas S, Alt-Epping B. Advance care planning in severe COPD: it is time to engage with the future. ERJ Open Research 2018;4(1):9.

18. Jabbarian LJ, Zwakman M, van der Heide A, et al. Advance care planning for patients with chronic respiratory diseases: a systematic review of preferences and practices. Thorax 2018;73(3):222–30.

19. Tripodoro VA, De Vito EL. What does end stage in neuromuscular diseases mean? Key approach-based transitions. Curr Opin Support Palliat Care 2015;9(4):361–8.

20. Murray L, Butow PN, White K, et al. Advance care planning in motor neuron disease: a qualitative study of caregiver perspectives. Palliat Med 2016; 30(5):471–8.

21. Rantala HA, Leivo-Korpela S, Kettunen S, et al. Survival and end-of-life aspects among subjects on long-term noninvasive ventilation. European Clinical Respiratory Journal 2021;8(1):1840494.

22. Smith TA, Disler RT, Jenkins CR, et al. Perspectives on advance care planning among patients recently requiring non-invasive ventilation for acute respiratory failure: a qualitative study using thematic analysis. Palliat Med 2017;31(6):566–74.

23. Smith TA, Kim M, Piza M, et al. Specialist respiratory physicians' attitudes to and practice of advance care planning in COPD. A pilot study. Respir Med 2014;108(6):935–9.

24. Reinke LF, Fasolino T, Sullivan DR. Goals of care and end-of-life communication needs of persons with chronic respiratory disease. Curr Opin Support Palliat Care 2023;17(4):283–9.

25. Bausewein C, Currow DC, Johnson MJ, editors. Palliative care in respiratory disease, vol. 73. Plymouth, UK: European Respiratory Society; 2016. p. 246.

26. Apatira L, Boyd EA, Malvar G, et al. Hope, truth, and preparing for death: perspectives of surrogate decision makers. Ann Intern Med 2008;149(12):861–8.

27. Dingfield LE, Kayser JB. Integrating advance care planning into practice. Chest 2017;151(6):1387–93.

28. Shalowitz DI, Garrett-Mayer E, Wendler D. The Accuracy of surrogate decision makers: a systematic review. Arch Intern Med 2006;166(5):493–7.

29. Schmidt TA, Hickman SE, Tolle SW, et al. The Physician Orders for Life-Sustaining Treatment program: Oregon emergency medical technicians' practical experiences and attitudes. J Am Geriatr Soc 2004; 52(9):1430–4.

30. Antonaglia C, Garuti G, Torregiani C. Management of patients with neuromuscular disorders and acute respiratory failure. Shortness of Breath 2014;3(4): 181–9.

31. Morélot-Panzini C, Perez T, Sedkaoui K, et al. The multidimensional nature of dyspnoea in amyotrophic lateral sclerosis patients with chronic respiratory failure: Air hunger, anxiety and fear. Respir Med 2018; 145:1–7.

32. Vrijsen B, Buyse B, Belge C, et al. Noninvasive ventilation improves sleep in amyotrophic lateral sclerosis: a prospective Polysomnographic study. J Clin Sleep Med 2015;11(05):559–66.

33. Janssens JP, Michel F, Schwarz EI, et al. Long-term mechanical ventilation: recommendations of the Swiss society of Pulmonology. Respiration 2020; 1–36.

34. Bourke SC, Tomlinson M, Williams TL, et al. Effects of non-invasive ventilation on survival and quality of life in patients with amyotrophic lateral sclerosis: a randomised controlled trial. Lancet Neurol 2006; 5(2):140–7.

35. Passamano L, Taglia A, Palladino A, et al. Improvement of survival in Duchenne muscular dystrophy: retrospective analysis of 835 patients. Acta Myol 2012;121–5.

36. Wilson E, Lee JS, Wenzel D, et al. The Use of mechanical ventilation support at the end of life in motor neurone disease/amyotrophic lateral sclerosis: a scoping review. Brain Sci 2022;12(9).

37. Association for Palliative Medicine of Great Britain and Ireland. Withdrawal of Assisted Ventilation at the Request of a Patient with Motor Neurone Disease, Available at: https://apmonline.org/wp-content/uploads/2016/03/Guidance-with-logos-updated-210316.pdf (Accessed 22 October 2023), 2015.

38. Chatwin M, Gonçalves M, Gonzalez-Bermejo J, et al. 252nd ENMC international workshop: Developing best practice guidelines for management of mouthpiece ventilation in neuromuscular disorders. March 6th to 8th 2020, Amsterdam, The Netherlands. Neuromuscul Disord 2020;30(9): 772–81.

39. Faull C, Rowe Haynes C, Oliver D. Issues for palliative medicine doctors surrounding the withdrawal of non-invasive ventilation at the request of a patient with motor neurone disease: a scoping study. BMJ Support Palliat Care 2014; 4(1):43–9.

40. Raveling T, Vonk J, Struik FM, et al. Chronic non-invasive ventilation for chronic obstructive pulmonary disease. Cochrane Database Syst Rev 2021; 8(8):CD002878.

41. Faes K, De Frène V, Cohen J, et al. Resource Use and health care Costs of COPD patients at the end of life: a systematic review. J Pain Symptom Manage 2016;52(4):588–99.

42. Yarra P, Annangi S. Early integration of palliative care in chronic obstructive pulmonary disease (COPD) is warranted based on symptom burden and quality of life. Evid Base Nurs 2020;24(4): 130.

43. Pihlaja H, Rantala H, Leivo-Korpela S, et al. Specialist palliative care Consultation for patients with Nonmalignant pulmonary diseases: a retrospective study. Palliat Med Rep 2023;4(1): 108–15.

44. Janssens J-P, Weber C, Herrmann FR, et al. Can early introduction of palliative care limit Intensive care, emergency and hospital Admissions in patients with severe chronic obstructive pulmonary disease? A pilot Randomized study. Respiration 2019; 97(5):406–15.

45. Caneiras C, Jácome C, Moreira E, et al. A qualitative study of patient and carer experiences with home respiratory therapies: long-term oxygen therapy and home mechanical ventilation. Pulmonology 2022;28(4):268–75.

46. Ribeiro C, Jácome C, Oliveira P, et al. Patients experience regarding home mechanical ventilation in an outpatient setting. Chron Respir Dis 2022;19. 14799731221137082.

47. Sullivan DR, Kim H, Gozalo PL, et al. Trends in noninvasive and invasive mechanical ventilation among Medicare Beneficiaries at the end of life. JAMA Intern Med 2021;181(1):93–102.

48. Smith TA, Davidson PM, Lam LT, et al. The use of non-invasive ventilation for the relief of dyspnoea in exacerbations of chronic obstructive pulmonary disease; a systematic review. Respirology 2012;17(2): 300–7.

49. Smith TA, Agar M, Jenkins CR, et al. Experience of acute noninvasive ventilation-insights from 'Behind the Mask': a qualitative study. BMJ Support Palliat Care 2019;9(1):e11.

50. Smith TA, Ingham JM, Jenkins CR. Respiratory failure, noninvasive ventilation, and symptom burden: an observational study. J Pain Symptom Manage 2019;57(2):282–289 e1.

51. Maddocks M, Lovell N, Booth S, et al. Palliative care and management of troublesome symptoms for people with chronic obstructive pulmonary disease. Lancet 2017;390(10098):988–1002.

52. Raveling T, Bladder G, Vonk JM, et al. Improvement in hypercapnia does not predict survival in COPD patients on chronic noninvasive ventilation. Int J Chron Obstruct Pulmon Dis 2018;13: 3625–34.

53. Pitre T, Abbasi S, Su J, et al. Home high flow nasal cannula for chronic hypercapnic respiratory failure in COPD: a systematic review and meta-analysis. Respir Med 2023;219:107420.

54. Zhang L, Wang Y, Ye Y, et al. Comparison of high-flow nasal cannula with Conventional oxygen therapy in patients with hypercapnic chronic obstructive pulmonary disease: a systematic review and meta-analysis. Int J Chron Obstruct Pulmon Dis 2023;18: 895–906.

55. Weinreich UM, Storgaard LH. A Real-life study of Combined treatment with long-term non-invasive ventilation and high flow nasal cannula in patients with end-stage chronic obstructive lung disease. J Clin Med 2023;12:4485.

56. Spicuzza L, Schisano M. High-flow nasal cannula oxygen therapy as an emerging option for respiratory failure: the present and the future. Ther Adv Chronic Dis 2020;11:1–15.

57. Swan F, Newey A, Bland M, et al. Airflow relieves chronic breathlessness in people with advanced disease: an exploratory systematic review and meta-analyses. Palliat Med 2019;33(6):618–33.

58. Ekstrom M, Nilsson F, Abernethy AA, et al. Effects of opioids on breathlessness and exercise capacity in chronic obstructive pulmonary disease. A systematic review. Ann Am Thorac Soc 2015;12(7): 1079–92.

59. Ekstrom M, Ferreira D, Chang S, et al. Effect of Regular, Low-dose, Extended-release Morphine on chronic breathlessness in chronic obstructive pulmonary disease: the BEAMS Randomized clinical trial. JAMA 2022;328(20):2022–32.

60. Simon ST, Higginson IJ, Booth S, et al. Benzodiazepines for the relief of breathlessness in advanced malignant and non-malignant diseases in adults. Cochrane Database Syst Rev 2016;10(10): CD007354.

61. Higginson IJ, Wilcock A, Johnson MJ, et al. Randomised, double-blind, multicentre, mixed-methods, dose-escalation feasibility trial of mirtazapine for better treatment of severe breathlessness in

advanced lung disease (BETTER-B feasibility). Thorax 2020;75(2):176–9.

62. Ekstrom M, Ahmadi Z, Bornefalk-Hermansson A, et al. Oxygen for breathlessness in patients with chronic obstructive pulmonary disease who do not qualify for home oxygen therapy. Cochrane Database Syst Rev 2016;11(11):CD006429.

63. Choi PJ, Murn M, Turner R, et al. Continuing noninvasive ventilation during amyotrophic lateral sclerosis-related hospice care is medically, Administratively, and Financially feasible. Am J Hosp Palliat Care 2021;38(10):1238–41.

64. Faull C, Wenzel D. Mechanical ventilation withdrawal in motor neuron disease: an evaluation of practice. BMJ Support Palliat Care 2020;12(e6): e752–8.

65. Lafferty M, Dunford M, Green H, et al. Evaluation of a 'level of dependency withdrawal of NIVs framework' in end-of-life respiratory failure patients. Eur Respir J 2023;62(suppl 67). PA4024.

66. Sennfalt S, Kläppe U, Thams S, et al. Dying from ALS in Sweden: clinical status, setting, and symptoms. Amyotroph Lateral Scler Frontotemporal Degener 2023;24(3–4):237–45.

Moving?

Make sure your subscription moves with you!

To notify us of your new address, find your **Clinics Account Number** (located on your mailing label above your name), and contact customer service at:

Email: journalscustomerservice-usa@elsevier.com

800-654-2452 (subscribers in the U.S. & Canada)
314-447-8871 (subscribers outside of the U.S. & Canada)

Fax number: 314-447-8029

Elsevier Health Sciences Division
Subscription Customer Service
3251 Riverport Lane
Maryland Heights, MO 63043

*To ensure uninterrupted delivery of your subscription, please notify us at least 4 weeks in advance of move.

Printed and bound by CPI Group (UK) Ltd, Croydon, CR0 4YY

08/05/2025

01864751-0017